Contents

KU-497-557

Tables

Illustration

1000324888

1 00 032788 5

FOOD POLICY REVIEW 2

H... T... useholds
Stress
ues

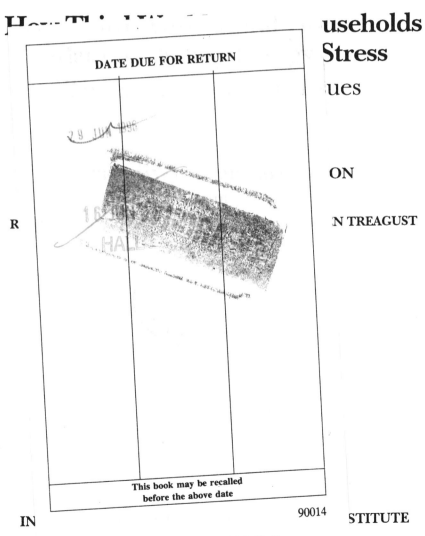

DATE DUE FOR RETURN

This book may be recalled
before the above date

90014

ON

R N TREAGUST

IN STITUTE

WASHINGTON, D.C.

Copyright 1994 International Food Policy
Research Institute.

All rights reserved. Sections of this report may
be reproduced without the express permission of
but with acknowledgment to the International
Food Policy Research Institute.

Library of Congress Cataloging-
in-Publication Data

Payne, Philip.
  How third world rural households adapt to
dietary energy stress : the evidence and the
issues / Philip Payne and Michael Lipton.
     p.   cm. — (Food policy review ; 2)
  Includes bibliographical references (p. 112).
  ISBN 0-89629-501-X
    1. Malnutrition—Developing   countries.
2. Adaptation (Physiology)—Developing countries. I. Lipton, Michael. II. Title. III. Series.

RA645.N87P39   1994   94-17153
616.3'9'0091724—dc20   CIP

Foreword

Recent IFPRI research has explored the effects of technical change and commercialization on the nutritional status of poor and often ill-nourished people. Even when incomes increase, household energy intakes and nutritional status are often little affected. This suggests that many poor people have ways of "adapting" to dietary energy stress and that they readjust to changes in the level of stress in complex ways.

Clearly, individuals have to respond in some way when food intake falls short of normal energy needs. The shortage may last for a day or a lifetime; the causes may vary from the physiological change of pregnancy to a seasonal labor peak. The response strategy may be biological: adults' weight may change; children's growth and final size may be altered. Behaviorally, working hours or methods may change. Socially, patterns of specialization or work-sharing may be modified. Which responses are likely, and for whom? Which are harmful, and how? Which are adaptive?

At the extremes, there is no disagreement among researchers. Severe undernourishment often kills; moderate fat loss by otherwise healthy adults is harmless—even beneficial. In between these extremes, however, there is intense controversy. Does mild stunting of children—a common response to energy stress—produce adults who are permanently disadvantaged, or simply "small but healthy"? Can people respond to acute stress just by reducing their metabolic rate? Are some responses adaptive, but only at costs that are unacceptable?

Crucial policy choices may depend on getting the right answers. Who needs what sort of help to cope with threatened energy stress? Are some forms of intervention counterproductive, negating natural adaptive mechanisms? Does concentration on the more severely stressed or most vulnerable leave the remainder exposed to less conspicuous forms of hunger, compelled to adapt in painful, irreversible ways?

In this volume, Philip Payne and Michael Lipton review the biological and social-science literature on the nature, sources, and types of energy stress, and the biological and behavioral adjustments displayed by individuals, households, and social groups. Many of the controversies can be resolved, and all can be clarified, by distinguishing clearly among sources and durations of stress, among diverse meanings attached to terms such as adaptation, and between the implications of a single desirable level and of a range of energy requirements. The authors emphasize the central questions of how humans respond to environmental stresses, and they attempt to embed the biology firmly in the behavioral context, especially that of rural developing areas.

Per Pinstrup-Andersen
Director General

Acknowledgments

We gratefully acknowledge comments from Harold Alderman, George Beaton, Jere Behrman, Anna Ferro-Luzzi, Maarten Immink, Philip James, John Mellor, Stephen Vosti, and John Waterlow; research collaboration from the National Institute of Nutrition, Hyderabad, India; and financial support from the Economic and Social Committee for Overseas Research, Overseas Development Administration, United Kingdom. None of these commentators and institutions, nor IFPRI, is necessarily in agreement with the judgments we have made.

Philip Payne
Michael Lipton

1

Summary

Two basic questions are addressed in this review. What are the biological and behavioral mechanisms used by individuals, households, or larger groups in adapting to the challenge of different sources, intensities, and durations of energy stress? And, given that successful adaptation implies only that an individual's chances of surviving to contribute to the inheritance of future generations are improved or maintained, what are the counterbalancing costs and who suffers most from them?

In the standard model of undernutrition, a source, such as a bad harvest, leads to energy stress, that is, deficient calorie intake, and in turn to bodily strain, such as stunting, followed by resultant damage, such as reduced IQ. Yet most statistical work, seeking to relate this damage to falls in household income per person, for example, achieves very low degrees of explanation. Why? First, there are too many uncertain links in the chain: lower income, unaltered household size, reduced total outlay, reduced food outlay, fewer calories, unchanged requirements, transmission to vulnerable household members, bad outcomes. Second, for each link, the model assumes the worst: either a harmful response, behavioral or biological, or none. Third, the model assumes the need for a fixed desirable level of individual energy intake relative to requirements: keeping within a range is not good enough.

This report, which reviews the evidence that there are types of persons, households, and situations for which adaptation to energy stress is achieved with low cost, tends to reject these gloomy assumptions. Organisms, including human individuals, families, and communities, make appropriate responses to energy stress through the various stages of the source-stress-strain-damage sequence. Like plants threatened with disease, some humans or groups threatened with energy stress can avoid the threat, repartition structures or activities to reduce its impact, resist that impact, or accept it but tolerate some damage. The responses themselves may be biological or behavioral and are often hierarchical (the less-damaging appearing earlier), but may also be integrated, involving several small adjustments at once. In exploring what sorts of people (families, groups) make various responses to energy stress, the guiding concepts of the review are adaptation and acceptability. A response is adaptive, or an adaptation, only if it increases the probability—given energy stress—of survival through the period of producing, and supporting to adulthood, viable and fertile offspring. An adaptive response is in addition acceptable only if it does not cause ethically unacceptable levels of pain or loss of functioning. In asking what response is acceptable or adaptive, a distinction is made here—for example, in the particular context of stunting—between the source of stress, the process of strain (of child growth retardation), and the possibility of damaging outcome in addition to reduced adult size.

Responses to energy stress are examined here along three time scales. First, the life-cycle of personal growth and development features a steadily reducing plasticity and reversibility of response to energy stress as the individual ages; intergenerational mother-to-child transmission of reduced size as a response, via womb size and metabolic regulation during pregnancy and lactation; and Darwinian selection, reflected in small but persistent and significant differences in mean body size among ethnic groups, which have selected against genes conferring undesirable responses to distinct conditions of energy (and climatic) stress and variability. Second, the household cycle changes response to energy stress as the worker/dependent ratio changes, but is itself surprisingly adjustable as families join or split under energy stress to exploit economies or diseconomies of scale. Third, the seasonal environmental cycle often induces adjustments in seasonal rates of conception to reduce energy stress upon mother or infant; in unexpected bad years, there is a hierarchy of responses to energy stress.

Reduced inputs, increased expenditure, and less-efficient conversion—the three modes in which energy stress impinges on people—are reviewed. Reduced energy inputs through sharpened poverty are all too familiar, but they also often arise from anorexia after infection, or because weaning gruels are too dilute or are offered in otherwise stressful situations. Worsened food energy retention (in dysentery or schistosomiasis) also in effect reduces inputs. Increased energy expenditure is a limited source of stress because the resting metabolic rate (RMR) comprises 50-75 percent of requirements. Recent evidence downgrades the role of pregnancy and lactation in energy stress. High altitude and temperatures outside the thermoneutral range produce intergenerational adaptations, though not necessarily free of cost. Decreased conversion efficiency—for example, as it becomes impaired by deficiencies of vitamin B (or perhaps other micronutrients)—can also cause energy stress.

The adaptiveness and acceptability of biological and behavioral adjustments are also considered. Biological processes include, first, changes in body or organ size and composition. Reduced child growth or adult weight is the commonest single adjustment. The data show that such reduction can generate very large "savings" in energy requirements, hence, for example, cumulative stunting can greatly reduce the risks of adult wasting. Mild early growth retardation may well be adaptive in most cases; poor children frequently become small adults, but they should not be judged malnourished by inappropriate standards, the achievement of which would not improve adaptation to environment. The final state—moderately smaller modal adults—is often acceptable, that is, it causes no significant pain or loss of functioning. However, the process of becoming small through childhood hunger or infection or both is normally unacceptable even if it is too mild to perceptibly increase the risks to life or functioning. Catch-up after the first two years is seldom complete. Even mild to moderate stunting persisting after that time may signal unhappiness or pain, but the balance of evidence is that it probably does not signal increased death risk, reduced resistance to infection, or worsened cognitive performance. Adult work capacity is somewhat reduced if measured by VO_2max, but not by actual VO_2 per kilogram—in most respects a more relevant measure.

Controversy still surrounds the second type of biological adaptation: the extent to which energy stress induces changes in the energy cost of resting metabolism in specific tissues. Interethnic differences of 10-15 percent in group mean RMR per kilogram are common; within ethnic groups, interpersonal differences of 10-15 percent induced by experimental energy stress are also common, but much larger ones have been found only in occasional nonreplicated studies or when accompanied by unacceptable side effects. The differences partly reflect "frozen," probably genetic, RMR accommodation to energy stress levels. Also, there is some evidence of 2-8 percent intrapersonal day-to-day variation in RMRs in response to energy stress. However, all this is hard to separate from other responses to energy stress: size or composition changes; declines in thermogenesis after subsequent exposure to cold, emotion, hormonal change, food, or infections; or rises in thermodynamic efficiency of conversion of dietary energy. All these responses to energy stress are feasible in principle. However, in field as distinct from laboratory conditions, substantial effects are seen only in pregnant and lactating women. Even then, the magnitude and pattern of response show major differences related to cultural or ethnic factors. Basic and applied research to establish the extent, causality, Darwinian variability, and possible "cost" and acceptability of such biological responses to energy stress is, literally, vital. In addition, it is necessary to learn whether they can be initiated or inhibited by particular behaviors (for example, rest in pregnancy or extra B vitamins). Major new policy instruments against nutritional damage might be an outcome of such research.

Overall, however, research strategies should recognize that behavioral responses to energy stress are probably much more important (commoner, larger, and more policy-influenced) than—and can remove the need, or even the capacity, for—biological responses. People often respond to stress periods via reduced energy expenditure: doing each task more slowly, or shifting rest or lighter tasks into such times. However, such responses to energy stress are usually available to the vulnerable poor, who are dependent on daily work for food, only to the extent that they are able to shift the tasks of food acquisition toward more energy-intensive or easily gathered foods or toward less-vulnerable household members. Ergonomic adaptations, that is, substitution of uncomfortable for energetic work by adults and reduction of play by children tend to be higher-cost (less "acceptable") adaptations.

The evidence on who is stressed, who adapts, and at what costs is summarized here, and conclusions and recommendations for further research are presented. Landlessness is correlated with risk of energy stress only where land is worth having, but becoming landless often doubly increases energy stress, raising expenditure (in job search) while at the same time reducing intake. Preagricultural hunter-gatherer populations offer striking examples of successful adaptation to often-severe energy stress, but at high cost to economic growth and perhaps to other components of well-being. Settled rural groups are usually more stressed than urban groups, but rural-urban migration (like agricultural settlement) carries new risks of energy stress that precedes learned responses; long-term migrants, however, usually show fewer signs of energy stress than the locally born. Most evidence suggests that only the extremely poor tend to increase energy intake substantially in response to income increases. But before it can be concluded that other people perceive themselves as adapted, more information is needed about how energy expenditures are related to changes or differences in income and energy intake.

2

Introduction

Precise Requirements
or Adaptive Ranges?

This report deals primarily with people living in rural areas of developing countries. The focus of concern is with those who suffer the various detrimental effects of low food consumption. To understand their plight, however, it is sometimes helpful to look also at a control group—people who are apparently similar in relevant ways to those harmed by low food consumption, yet somehow avoid or reduce the ill effects.

The study concentrates upon those particular ill effects that would be removed if the intake of energy alone were to be increased to some higher level, even with no addition in other nutrient intakes, for a sufficiently long period. Along with such undernutrition, other forms of malnutrition (such as specific deficiencies of micronutrients) exist in these areas, and furthermore, both forms exist outside the rural sector. However, there is abundant evidence, not recounted here, that the greatest extent of food insecurity, and hence the greatest potential for undernutrition, is to be found in the rural areas of developing countries.

The standard picture of such undernutrition is roughly as follows. First, there is a variety of causes or sources of stress in the external environment: ill health, absent or wrong knowledge about what constitutes a safe and adequate diet, and maldistribution of resources or tasks within households. However, it is frequently claimed that the primary source of stress—whether or not in association with other causes—is household income per adult-equivalent that is insufficient to acquire enough food to cover household energy requirements, given (1) the energy that must be expended to obtain income, and (2) the income required to prepare food (for example, to buy fuel) and to meet unavoidable nonfood needs.

Second is the stress itself. This can take the form of a low (or falling) energy intake, a high (or rising) requirement, or an inadequate (or worsening) capacity to convert food intake into energy requirement. According to the standard picture, the upshot is always the same: food intake, for a significant period, falls below the food requirement for maintenance of body weight in adults (or adequate increase of weight in children), protection of the body against illness, and full discharge of physical and mental requirements.

5

Third, such stress creates strains within the household. The strains are seen as physiological or biochemical changes in the bodies of the individual members. They are affected, in part, by changes in the distribution of food within the household. The strains are liable to prevail as long as the household's energy intake falls short of its previous, or of desired, levels of energy expenditure.

Fourth, the result of strain may or may not be damage. Usually, in adults, body weights or levels of physical activity or both are reduced. In children, growth is sometimes slower than it might be. Even if some part of that outcome is avoided (for example, by reducing energy expenditure below desirable levels) or tolerated, the upshot may be curtailed mental or physical functioning. This is further assumed (in the standard picture) to lead to depleted economic performance and, in more severe or prolonged cases—especially when it happens to very young infants—to increased illness, mental retardation, or even death.

Such results certainly happen in particular cases, during severe or prolonged undernutrition. However, many observations have cast doubt on the general applicability of the above "standard picture" to more moderate or briefer episodes of undernutrition. Consider the most well known and widely tested version, the link between household income and infant nutrition. When a household's income per adult-equivalent falls too low to meet the desirable and normal levels of energy expenditure, it is likely to cause (1) reduced consumption outlay, leading in turn to (2) reduced outlay on food, (3) reduced energy availability, (4) reduced energy consumption relative to (less than proportionately reduced) expenditure, (5) the passing on of a significant and perhaps even disproportionate part of this reduction to vulnerable infants within the household, (6) substantial setbacks for these infants in height-for-age, and (7) harmful outcomes in terms of illness, reduced mental or physical capacity, or increased risk of death.

At each of the seven points in this chain at which a behavioral or biological alternative is open, the above sequence of events assumes the worst: either no response or a damaging one. Since less-harmful alternatives often exist, it is not surprising that the linkages between (1) and (7)—between income inadequacy or decline, on the one hand, and bad outcomes for nutrition-related functioning of infants (or anyone else), on the other—are weak, except in extreme cases. This is partly because some households are better than others at preventing such outcomes; partly because of variables not in the equations; and partly because of random events, such as which people catch an infection. For all these reasons, regression equations that estimate the dependence of the nutrition-related health status of infants on income, or on several other "standard picture" variables such as household size and structure, health environment, and nutrition education, typically yield r-squared values as low as 0.1, even though the effect of each explanatory variable is usually in the expected direction and often statistically highly significant (see, for example, Bouis and Haddad 1990, 54; Behrman and Deolalikar 1988, 660-672, and references therein; von Braun, Hotchkiss, and Immink 1989, 85.)

Clearly, some households and some household members are managing to avoid, redirect, or reduce the damaging effects upon health or behavior that are often associated with poverty or other sources of stress. This happens even under circumstances where damage does occur in many other households that are not, apparently, any poorer or otherwise more vulnerable than those that escape.

There may well be hidden costs to the households that limit damage, though an onus of proof is surely upon those who claim that such costs exist. Even if these costs are absent in some households, that need not mean that many other households or individuals could be expected to cope with a similar kind or level of stress without cost, if only they were more knowledgeable or clever. Nor need it mean that the households able to deal with a particular stress at fairly low cost (whether by avoiding strain or by containing it or its effects) could deal with more severe or prolonged dietary energy stress caused by the same source. For example, a household that can endure a 10 percent cut in dietary energy intake for three weeks without permanent damage might not be able to do so for five weeks, or even for three weeks with a 15 percent cut. Even if a 10 percent cut in energy intake for three weeks were manageable, a different time-distribution of the same energy shortfall—for example, a 20 percent cut for one and a half weeks—might not be. Nor might even the "same" size *and* distribution of stress from a different source: for example, a three-week 10 percent rise in requirements with no change in intake. For pregnant women, a reduction of energy stress via extra rest is apparently better than an "identical" reduction via extra energy intake (Briend 1984).

There is no implication that, if each of the above stresses can be handled with no lasting damage, it could be presumed that the source of stress was not a bad thing, or that (say) the household suffering from it on grounds of low income was not "really" poor. Acute hunger, or overwork at low energy intake, is nasty in itself even if it has no (or containable) consequences for bodily or mental state or function. Further, even if acute hunger (as well as dietary energy stress) is avoided, the household may remain poor in other respects than shortage of energy.

However, it would be a major advance to be able to identify the types of persons, households, or situations that made for relatively low-cost outcomes to various stresses that in other circumstances produced severe strains and damaging outcomes. At best, lessons from the former circumstances could be used to reduce damage in the latter. But suppose that this is not possible: for example, that the capacity to increase ergonomic efficiency, and thereby to adapt to seasonal falls in intake alongside high work needs, turns out to be almost wholly genetic. Even that disappointing result would provide policymakers in developing countries, who (notwithstanding food surpluses in the West) face severe constraints on their capacity to provide basic foods and health services, with useful guidance for the effective allocation of such resources. For example, programs of food relief or health improvement could go first to areas where at-risk groups are less able, for genetic reasons, to increase ergonomic efficiency and thereby to adapt to seasonal strain or to resulting bodily stress, while programs providing chances to earn more income (even in the stressed season) could go first to areas where at-risk groups are better able to adapt. See for example, the section in

Chapter 4, "Changes in Specific Metabolic Rates of Tissues: Metabolic Adaptation," and references therein.

This review outlines the relevant evidence on stresses, strains, and low-cost and high-cost adaptations. But before the problems are introduced, two worries should be disposed of. First, economists may worry that this approach, by seeking to "teach" the poor to subsist at lower levels of income and nutrition, somehow distracts from the need to increase their productivity and welfare. The function of social policy, including nutritional policy, is to increase human capabilities, not to raise passive satisfaction by lowering human activity or output, with the possible outcome that "the underdog learns to bear the burden so well that . . . discontent is replaced by acceptance . . . suffering and anger by cheerful endurance" (Sen 1984, 309). However, greater human robustness under stress might result from a better understanding of the essential conditions for coping, and this robustness in turn could increase the capability to cope, besides reducing deaths or suffering of people still left vulnerable to even higher levels of stress. Such robustness, especially where the authorities are not very concerned with poverty reduction, should help the poor in their economic and political performance.

Second, nutritionists may worry that an adaptationist approach implies undue or premature acceptance of the view (Sukhatme and Margen 1982) that some or all persons can substantially and costlessly reduce their energy requirements as a response to energy stress; for example, by reducing their rate of energy expenditure per unit of body weight at rest (basal metabolic rate [BMR] per kilogram). While most authorities agree that some such metabolic adaptation exists, there is no agreement about either the average extent or the range of variation of individual capacity to respond in this way without incurring serious damage either in the short or long run. The study concludes, from current evidence, that this will turn out to be considerably less than the downward adaptations of BMR per kilogram of around 20 percent demonstrated by Keys et al. (1950) in conditions of semistarvation; under such conditions, the accompanying side effects on the subjects could not be regarded as harmless. There are, however, many kinds of responses, other than via involuntary changes in BMR per kilogram, that can legitimately be regarded as adaptations to dietary energy stress. Sometimes, as discussed later, such responses are quite large. They are seldom, if ever, costless, but the jury is still out on whether they are low-cost. Certainly they often represent the "least evil."

The general conclusion of this study is that, just as there is a wide variety of causes or sources of energy stress, so there is a variety of responses open to individuals, households, or larger social groups. Moreover, not only does undernutrition usually have multiple and connected causes, the total response itself is commonly both complex and strategic. The elements of that strategy may be partly sequential. There may well be an ordering of the functions that are to change under energy stress: work, weight, or whatever. Such an ordering observes a set of rules, probably inherited (genetically or socially), about degrees of indispensability of different biological functions, or the social worth of different individuals or capabilities. At any given time during the evolution of the strategy, the mix of different kinds of biological and behavioral responses will also reflect trade-offs derived from inheritance of characteristics and from past experience.

Plan of Work

In attempting to integrate the whole range of social and biological aspects there is a danger of giving an impression of a disordered complexity. Therefore, the remainder of this chapter is devoted to developing a conceptual framework.

The different time scales over which stress may operate to produce the resulting strain experienced, or damage suffered, are examined in Chapter 3. First is the biological time scale, covering the life span of the individual from birth through the life cycle, but also extending to intergenerational effects—indeed, to effects transmitted across the many generations involved in the molding of characters through natural selection. Second is the time scale of the household cycle, from couple formation (in the nuclear household) to death of the widow or widower. Third is the environmental time scale of seasons, years, and cycles that may impose stress affecting many individuals and induce strain in some or all (and costly consequences in a subset of those who are strained).

This is followed by a discussion in Chapter 4 of the different ways in which energy stress operates upon individuals—essentially, through lowered intakes, increases in expenditure, or reduced efficiency of conversion of food into desired "outputs."

Two broad categories of responses to stress, biological and behavioral, are then examined in Chapters 5 and 6. For example, for slower child growth considered as a biological reaction to smaller dietary energy intake, or for the behavioral reaction of altered tasks, an attempt is made to sort out adaptations from other responses, and low-cost or "acceptable" adaptations from others.

Building on the results of this classification, evidence is presented in Chapter 7 as to which groups of rural people in developing countries (by location, poverty, age, sex, and so forth) are stressed and which of these seem able to adapt at low cost, either by avoiding strain or by accommodating to it.

Adapting to What?
Source, Stress, Strain, Damage

One important aim of this inquiry into nutritional adaptation is to clarify the controversy that has surrounded the definition and use of nutrient requirements. In particular, it is necessary to estimate the capacity (if any) of various people or groups for adaptation, at low cost, to varying degrees, durations, and concomitants of nutritional stress, such as a shortfall of dietary energy intake below normal requirements for the maintenance of fitness.

The words "adaptation" and "fitness" are used by evolutionists to denote precisely defined concepts but have been redefined of late by many others to cover a range of meanings, some colloquial rather than scientific. This has been due in part to the justified concern of both social and natural scientists with the issues of hunger and deprivation. For example, some people use the term "adaptive response" to describe one apparent upshot of dietary energy stress for whole populations—relatively small body size. Whether such a term is appropriate does not appear to be a scientific question. It is partly a matter of the subjective reaction of the listener or reader, and such a reaction tends to be highly emotive ("small but healthy" versus "tall Westerners who tell the South to stay small"). Therefore, it is necessary to clarify how such words will be used in this report.

The word "stress," in common usage, generally connotes something unpleasant (it is in fact a contracted form of "distress"): at best, something to be avoided; at worst, a threat to life or happiness. To an engineer or biologist, however, the word simply describes the forces or interactions between systems and their external environments. An animal, a piece of machinery, a colony of birds, or a building—all are constantly exposed to the stresses of various external forces applied to them, whether mechanical or otherwise. Thus, a building is stressed by the weight of its contents, or by the pressure of wind, or by the shock wave of an earthquake.

Other kinds of words are needed to describe how systems adjust to applied stresses. Beams bend, whole buildings tilt, animals hibernate, colonies migrate. The engineer uses these responses to quantify the "strain" in a system and will characterize the way a structure handles different levels of stress in terms of stress-strain relationships.

Evidently it is the nature and magnitude of these various adjustments or strains, taken together, that constitute the overall reaction to stress in a plant or animal and, combined with knowledge about the side effects and secondary results of the component adjustments, finally determine whether the outcome is assessed as good or bad. If the aim is to clarify the relationships between nutritional and other kinds of stresses in the environment and the responses that individuals and societies make to them, it is of the utmost importance to use words in a consistent way, especially to preserve the distinction between stress and response, which common usage tends to blur. Four possible components of the sequence of threat and reaction—the threat of undernutrition and the reaction by a preemptive strategy adopted by humans—are defined as follows:

The *source* of stress is the external agent capable of producing a high or increased level of energy requirement relative to energy intake; for example, a drought that threatens food supply (tending to reduce intake) or a season of especially hard work (tending to increase requirements).

The *stress* itself is the resulting energy imbalance arising from the high or increased level of energy requirements, or from the low or reduced level of either energy intake or food conversion efficiency, or from a combination of these.

The *strain* is one or more of the detectable, but in themselves not necessarily damaging, bodily signs of reaction to stress such as falls in weight, reduced child growth, or lower levels of response of the immune system to infections, together with changes in behavior such as work patterns and social interactions.

The *damage* from strain is the overall negative effect on mental or bodily condition, wellness, physical or social performance, or in extreme cases, survival prospects.

Can humans, households, or groups be said to "adapt" to any of these four parts of the sequence? Biologists generally use the word "adaptive" to describe responses or adjustments to environmental stress that, by accommodating the system to that stress, make a positive contribution toward fitness within the new environment: the individual or group is better able to cope with its new circumstances as a result of the responses it has made. While acknowledging the complexity of response to environmental stresses and the subtlety of the consequences of the physiological and behavioral changes that may be involved, evolutionary biologists are usually content to say that the net effects of these can be judged according to whether or not the outcome favors the fitness and hence survival of the genotype.

Faced with the proposition that some responses to nutritional stress should be regarded as adaptive, social and public health scientists have generally been unwilling to use this term on the grounds that it seems to imply some kind of success, even if only in a biological sense. We, they say, should not be willing to describe a human condition as successful when it is in fact the outcome of a process that succeeds through the barest survival of individuals (or, even worse, at the price of individual deaths, so that the only real success is the survival of the genotype).

For example, Beaton (1985, 221) writes, "The assertion that [because] humans can survive and function on intakes below current requirement estimates . . . there must be adaptation . . . is correct only if one is prepared to waive the definition of 'health' embodied in the original requirement estimate." This is true only if the word "adaptation" is used in a perfectionist, rather than an evolutionary, sense. In other contexts, the word has been subject to qualification of its meaning by coupling it with such terms as successful, cost-free, and pure. Besides adding to the confusion, this has tended to support the view of many health professionals that *any* detectable strain resulting from nutritional stress should be regarded as evidence of departure from a more desirable, perhaps optimal state—that is, as a priori evidence of malnutrition.

There is of course general agreement that there are *some* levels of stress that are excessive because they give rise to levels of strain that do significant damage, perhaps inconsistent with survival. Such responses, by definition, are not adaptive. Buildings distort to the point that doors and windows stick; or indeed the structure is taken beyond the yield point of some component, so that the stress-strain relationship is permanently changed to the extent that there is now a risk of catastrophic failure. Part of the current controversy, however, is about whether nutritional requirements should be based simply on the intakes needed to avoid such damage, and if so, how to agree on the kinds and levels of risk that should be so avoided. In the past, this controversy was about the amounts needed for the maintenance of some allegedly optimum state of nutritional health (in Beaton's terms, the definition of health embodied in the requirements estimate). Today most nutritionists would accept the concept of an adaptive range, within which different levels of stress can be accommodated without incurring significant risk to survival or reproductive performance.

Differences in the points at which two persons are placed on the range would be expected to arise through (1) variation between the modal members of two distinct populations, because different sets of environmental factors operating over time will produce different gene-environment equilibria; (2) interindividual variation, because people may need different amounts of energy for the same life-patterns even if they are identical in body size and composition (even though, as discussed in the following section, the extent of metabolic adaptations may be small); and (3) intraindividual variation, because the energy requirements of an individual may change over time (even holding weight and work constant) as that individual responds to changes of life-patterns or environment. While such variations are unlikely to be cost-free, no persuasive evidence is available that there exists a preferred, or optimum, point within the range. Moving toward any particular point, too, has costs. To specify an optimum, and seek to induce movement toward it, is therefore to seriously constrain choices in, and to reduce resources for, health planning.

Response, Adjustment, Adaptation, Acceptability

For the sake of consistency and clarity, the various ways in which the components of a system react to stress are referred to here as "adjustments" or, in the case of a whole organism or social group, as "responses." The word "adaptation," unless preceded by the adjective "acceptable," will be confined to its evolutionary sense. That is to say, it will be used in relation to responses to stress likely to have contributed in the past to "fitness," in the sense of increased or maintained probability, given the stress, of survival through the period of producing and supporting viable offspring. Adaptations are normally to a new maintainable steady state (until senescence), conservative of functions under threat, and sometimes, though not necessarily, reversible (Waterlow 1985). If conditions have, in the past, proved sufficiently likely to change in such a way that an individual's reversal of a previous adaptation contributes to fitness, then the capacity to reverse becomes a part of the adaptation.

For purposes of this review, it seems best to adhere to this restricted definition, which stems from the belief that comprehension of the nature and implications of the various possibly adaptive responses, biological or behavioral, and of the probable nature of the events that shaped those responses in the past, is essential to the improvement of an understanding of contemporary human energy needs and must precede any review of popular, or morally appropriate, judgments about acceptability.

It is necessary, of course, to consider the acceptability or otherwise of the various (alleged) forms and degrees of nutritional adaptation, given their role in contributing to biological fitness. The question of whether they have acceptable implications, either for the quality of life of the individuals affected or for the peace of mind of others aware of them, will be discussed in detail in Chapters 5 and 6. It is, however, worth stressing at once (in view of such contributions as Gopalan 1983) that all adaptations that lastingly reduce a person's human capability (Sen 1984, 309) are regarded as unacceptable; for example, those of a household that adapts to energy stress by withdrawing a child from school, let alone by so curtailing its growth or play that its adult potentials are significantly impaired.

However, the debate about acceptable adaptation can be narrowed down and is not usually a disagreement about values or norms. Many arguments about whether a given adaptation is acceptable would be resolved if agreement could be reached about the facts of how particular biological or behavioral processes and responses work. Furthermore, some arguments, such as those about whether small body size is an acceptable outcome of environmental stress, confuse two different things. As Beaton (1989) rightly emphasizes, levels of environmental stress to which infants are commonly exposed in poor communities are responsible for the process of becoming small and are generally not acceptable. Such levels of stress are sometimes traceable to food deprivation alone, but this is almost always associated with—indeed often preceded and sometimes caused by—other damaging events such as infections and diseases of childhood. These not only affect growth when they occur, but may also produce other long-lasting effects that increase the risk of failure of health and performance in adult life; but the process can often be halted or reversed. By contrast, the state of being small (the result of that process) is often harmless, sometimes contributes to fitness (that is, is adaptive), and once established is often wholly or largely irreversible after the first two or three years of life. This confusion is sustained by the common practice of referring to measurements of size or of growth retardation (anthropometric indicators) in children as indicators of current nutritional status, when in practice the etiology of smallness is much more complex than that simple description would imply. While shortness in a young infant may be an indicator that the process is happening, shortness in a school child is likely to mean no more than that it happened in the past.

There is good reason to conclude that smallness, that is, the state of being small, is sometimes adaptive. The significance of changes in body size as part of a strategy of response to energy stress will be considered later in more detail.

It remains to be seen whether smallness constitutes an acceptable adaptation. The viewpoint in this study is that it does so if and only if the children's mental and physical functioning through adulthood is unimpaired (as can be shown for nonwasted, moderate stunting; see the excellent and balanced review by Osmani [1988]). There is no unanimity over this, although again the argument is confused by semantics. For example, Waterlow (1985) cites evidence that small-for-age Indian boys "earn less money," and concludes that "the person who characterizes these children as adapted . . . is simply preempting a whole series of value judgments." However, this is the case only if "adapted" is taken to mean "adapted acceptably or at negligible cost or both." It is argued here that they are adapted (in a more restricted sense of the word) if and only if their smaller height-for-age, once achieved, does not harm their survival-and-reproduction prospects, given their likely food, work, and health conditions.

However, the much-debated issue of whether small can be beautiful (or healthy) cannot be resolved quite so easily. While almost all participants in these controversies (including the authors of this review) would agree that the processes of stress and deprivation involved in the generation of smallness are unacceptable in terms of human values, for the reasons already stated, it is of real practical importance to gain as much understanding as possible about the degree of acceptability or otherwise of the outcome of those processes. Beaton (1989) inclines toward the view that big is best on the grounds that, although moderate degrees of smallness are not known to be associated with any loss of functional capacity, they might nonetheless imply an unacceptable loss of potential for change; that is to say, a reduced ability of an individual to respond to new and possibly advantageous circumstances. This could be so—nobody knows. But loss of adaptive capacity is an important cost only if such capacity (1) is likely to be needed in future, (2) could as well be associated with nonadaptation as with adaptation, and (3) above all, might be occasioned by any irreversible response—for example, by one that led to greater tallness, just as well as by a height-retarding response. Tallness closes some options, shortness others. Thus, while the jury may remain out for some time on the empirical effects of height and weight on health and fitness to actual or potential environments and life-styles, there is no apparent reason to accept any a priori argument that "taller" must mean "more adaptable later," or otherwise "better."

It is an empirical issue, not a question of pure logic. Nor is it a question of sociomedical ethics. It is a caricature to claim, as some do (Messer 1986; Gopalan 1983; Dasgupta and Ray 1986, 633-34), that adaptation-optimists (for example, Seckler 1985 and Sukhatme 1961) generally want to define away undernutrition by statistical sleight-of-hand and to "accept" the status quo, namely, the absence of radical antipoverty policies and high risks of reduced human functioning due to undernutrition. It is equally a caricature to accuse adaptation-pessimists of seeking to maximize demand for nutritionists (or for food), or to deflect reform away from improving the control by the poor of assets and toward the more politically innocuous provision of food handouts.

Responses: Avoidance, Repartition, Resistance, Tolerance

In order to describe the sequence of causes and outcomes of stress, the terminology of construction engineering is borrowed to distinguish source, stress, strain, and damage. Borrowing from another subject, plant breeding, is also useful to introduce some terms that describe four different categories of adaptive response to disease.

Avoidance is typified in plants by growth in places, seasons, or years with relatively low risk, for example, of drought or attack by insects. *Repartitioning* describes the strategy of directing the threat or its consequences toward less vulnerable times or tissues (for example, leaves rather than roots), or toward some individual plants in a group whose members share a similar and relatively robust genetic constitution. *Resistance* consists of development or selection of characteristics or behaviors that ward off the threat (for example, secretion of a chemical that deters an insect pest). *Tolerance* implies the acceptance of some damage that is sufficiently small or reversible, or both, to be regarded as acceptable by the plant breeder.

What is acceptable involves judgments of value. If these responses are made by humans, rather than plants, then to the extent that people can choose (or alter the range of choice for others) among possible responses, there is inevitably some trading-off of costs and benefits. In practice in any specific situation, the outcome will reflect, in varying degree, some elements of "obligatory" responses originating from established evolutionary patterns, "traditional" responses in conformity with patterns of socioeconomic power or culture, and "voluntary" selection involving conscious evaluation of alternatives.

These four kinds of adaptive responses have their counterparts in those made by human individuals or groups in the face of a threat of undernutrition. Together with the four stages of challenge (source, stress, strain, damage), they can be set out as a diagram (Figure 1). Different responses to any particular stage of challenge can be reviewed by looking at the row for that stage in the diagram. For example, how might a person respond to a particular *source* of energy stress, that is, to a threat from that source to generate a stress? Suppose the source of stress is a reduction in wage rates or employment opportunities. An individual may respond by avoidance; for example, learning a new skill or moving to another location. Or the response might be to repartition the threat by spending less money on nonfood items or by shifting

Figure 1—Pattern of nutritional challenges and responses

		Sequence of Responses			
		Avoidance	Repartition-ing	Resistance	Tolerance
Stage of Challenge	Source				
	Stress	////			
	Strain	////	////		
	Damage	////	////	////	

Note: Hatched sections indicate that the response is not feasible for the stage of challenge.

unemployment to less stressful times of year. The individual might resist
the threat, that is, neutralize it, by purchasing cheaper food items, or
tolerate it by simply cutting down slightly on all expenditures and
accepting some resulting degree of hunger.

Suppose now that sufficient hunger has come about to cause energy
stress—if the pattern of intakes, food conversion efficiency, and expenditure on physical activities is unchanged. Avoidance is now ruled out. The
"stress" row in Figure 1 shows that the stress could be countered
through repartitioning—for example, by redirecting energy expenditure toward work through a reduction in the proportion spent on leisure
activities; through resisting—for example, by becoming more ergonomically efficient; or through tolerating, that is, by accepting the need to
make physiological response, which normally involves acceptance of
several small strains, none severe enough to cause serious damage.

Now suppose that the intake-activity pattern cannot be so changed
as to prevent significant *strain*. Both avoidance and repartitioning are
now by definition ruled out. However, the strain could be resisted by
reducing body weight or changing body composition to the point where
energy balance is restored (note that the presence of strain implies that
such repartitioning appears as resistance). Or the strain could be tolerated for a limited time; for example, body-fat reserves could be depleted
during a bad period in the expectation of repletion at a later time.

Finally, if permanent *damage* results—for example, as a consequence
of an unusually extended drought—the person might become permanently dependent on less physically demanding employment or upon
charity or state handouts. "Damage" implies that its tolerance is the only
remaining strategy; its limitation, to the extent possible, had already been
achieved as shown in earlier rows of Figure 1 (by resisting or tolerating
strain; resisting, tolerating, or repartitioning stress; and so forth).

The same sequence of threat-responses could be followed by a
household or a larger social group. Households can avoid seasonal
unemployment as a source of stress by a regular migration cycle. Or they
can repartition the source by separation into fixed and seasonally migra-
tory members. They might resist, by concentrating domestic and home
maintenance tasks into the slack season. Or they might tolerate, at the
expense of enduring a "hungry" season.

Looking along the stress row in Figure 1, seasonal restriction of food
to the extent that energy stress occurs (because total physical activity
cannot be curtailed without loss of production or income) could be
repartitioned by a household; for example, by maintaining the intakes of
those members able to sustain employment, at the expense of greater
stress for the remainder. Stress could be resisted by the reduction of
leisure or cultural exchanges, or by the specialization of appropriately
adapted household members in hard work at moderately low food
intakes, while others perform greatly reduced work at food intakes
closer to the resting metabolic rate (see Chapter 7).

Strain could be resisted by the temporary or permanent transfer of
nonproductive members to households of relatives, or tolerated as a little
strain for everyone in proportion to capacity to withstand it. However, if
too much strain has to be tolerated, someone in the household may suffer

damage: permanent, or substantial though temporary, loss of physical or mental capacity by some members, with consequent loss of income.[1] It remains feasible for a household to tolerate a limited degree of damage.

This classification has been found useful in reviewing the literature because it provides a framework within which the social and physiological adjustments can be seen together as components of an overall strategy of response. Wherever possible, the categories are sharply distinguished. However, it is clear that in any real situation the outcome is likely to be some combination—a little of several of the 10 options shown in Figure 1. The borderlines between physical threats—between source and stress, stress and strain, strain and damage—are not always clear-cut; neither are those between the organism's responses (whether behavioral or biological)—between avoidance and repartitioning, repartitioning and resistance, or resistance and tolerance. Also, it is not always clear-cut whether an organism's response is a low-cost adaptation that conserves all or almost all desirable features of human functions, an adaptation that fails to do so (and is for this reason generally regarded as unacceptable) although it does conserve fitness to survive,[2] or a failure to adapt.

All the hatched boxes in Figure 1 are necessarily (logically) empty for *all* initial row or column specifications. Other boxes may be contingently (empirically) empty for *some* specifications. For example, consider "avoidance of source." One important "source" of energy stress, malaria, cannot be avoided at all, in practice, by many communities. Also, the same *general* description of a particular row and column may, for two different *exact* specifications, lead to different box entries. For example, consider the row for the stress, "a deficit in energy intake relative to work done." The possible entries in the boxes for the "resistance" and "tolerance" columns will probably be quite different if the event causing the stress was (1) a fall in energy intake without a corresponding fall in expenditure, or (2) a rise in work done without a matching increment of food.

Finally, responses by animals, especially humans, to the sequence of challenges posed by undernutrition raise four linked issues:

- If one thinks of a single attribute of an individual animal, such as weight or length or peak work capacity, there is normally a range

---

[1] A commentator points out that a household's "resistance to strain" can take the form of withdrawing children from school because they are needed to gather food or because they are too hungry to perform properly at school or both. This is a clear case of an adaptation that is biologically "successful" but not acceptable in human terms. Indeed, couples, and especially girls who commence but do not complete primary education, produce at least as large completed families as those who do not go to school at all (World Bank 1984). On the relationship between anthropometry, amount and timing of schoolchild's and household's food intake, school performance, and final outcomes for the school child, see "Cognition" section in Chapter 5.

[2] Sometimes the changed biological response is acceptable, sometimes not. For example, the decision to continue with hard work despite seasonal energy stress may trigger increases in ergonomic (or perhaps metabolic) efficiency for some people, harmless weight loss for others, and serious damage to yet others. It would be very useful to know which people, or communities, fell into each category.

of values that a measurement of that attribute might assume, all of which are compatible with adaptive fitness. Over this range, functional impairment is sufficiently limited that there is no significant increase in the risk that the organism will not survive to, or procreate normally during, the reproductive period. If the value in a specific case is determined by gene-environment interaction,[3] the environment is subject to change, or if the organism is mobile among environments (as are animals, especially humans), then it is much likelier that there is a range of sufficient levels, over which that attribute supports survival of the adequately fit, rather than a single "optimizing" value, at which it favors survival of the fittest.

• As the borders of this range are approached, there is a hierarchy of responses across the Figure 1 diagram, normally involving ordering—avoidance before repartitioning before resistance, with tolerance the last resort—but sometimes disordering, complementarity, cumulation, or occlusion, or a combination of these.

Ordering. At the extremes, much safer or cheaper responses appear sooner. For example, at a given cost, an organism normally avoids a source of stress, rather than seeking to tolerate damage from strain (the "response of last resort" to prevent decline).

Disordering. A biological or behavioral response might be in some sense "less desirable" than a rejected alternative response. For example, children may go hungry in drought (Jodha 1975), or may be denied schooling so that they may earn or preserve energy (see footnote 1, p. 17), long before the household decisionmaker is prepared to sell an asset. There is a reluctance to overtly sacrifice long-run family well-being in order to feed or school the children adequately in the short run.

Complementarity. Often, several responses complement each other: trading down to cheaper food; deferral of strenuous tasks; task-specific slowing-down (usually involving increased ergonomic, though reduced economic, efficiency—see Chapter 6); avoidance of work where risk of infection is high; perhaps a little more metabolic efficiency.

Cumulation. Each response may be small, either because the physiological or thermodynamic constraints limit the extent to which a particular component of energy exchange can be altered, or because that component is a small fraction of the total. Yet three or four such responses may cumulate enough to balance the stress while avoiding unacceptable damage. See Table 1 for a very approximate summary of the main components of total daily

---

[3]Across generations, the possibility of the emergence among individuals of a range of values of some variable attribute that contributes to survival is increased if the genetic information, which controls the expression of that attribute, is distributed among several gene-pairs (especially if some of these are initially heterozygotes). That is because natural selection will then favor offspring that inherit the appropriate identical recessive(s) from each parent as well as those that inherit appropriate dominant gene(s).

Table 1—Energy intakes and outputs of 55-kilogram male Indian peasant

Item	Energy Category	Daily Kilocalories	Scope for Energy-Saving Adjustment
Intake equivalent to 780 grams of paddy	Gross energy content of food eaten Energy absorbed and metabolized	2,800 2,520	The 280 (2,800–2,520) kilocalories typically lost during digestion, absorption, and incomplete metabolism of food might be reduced by 15-20 percent. But if cheaper foods are used, these may be less efficiently absorbed.
Expenditure	Basal metabolic rate (BMR)	1,400	**Body-Weight Related** ~15 percent reduction if body weight reduced by 10 kilograms — **Metabolism Related** ~10 percent reduction of BMR independent of weight change
	Physical activity essential for sustaining life	380	~15 percent reduction in proportion to reduced BMR and body weight — ~10 percent saving due to reduced thermogenesis, diet regulated, work related, and stress related
	Physical activity essential for sustaining social participation	180	~15 percent reduction in proportion to reduced BMR and body weight
	Productive work	500	**Work Pattern and Work Efficiency** ~5-10 percent by ergonomic adjustments ~100 percent at cost of loss of income
	Leisure	60	100 percent

Note: These figures are entirely notional and are intended simply to provide a framework for what follows.

energy exchange for a moderately active adult male engaged in farm work and not currently suffering from energy stress.

Occlusion. One response (usually behavioral) may occlude another (usually biological), limiting or preventing its emergence or learning, or concealing its potential presence or size, or both. For example, if the adult male chooses to work less when his calorie intake falls, one cannot readily test whether—if he had instead chosen to maintain his prestress level of work—his ergonomic or metabolic efficiency would have risen. This is analogous to the frequent occlusion of horizontal resistance to disease in plant varieties that are bred for vertical resistance (Simmonds 1981, 265-267).

- Response may, as indicated, be biological or behavioral. Possibly adaptive biological responses include (1) "phenotypic plasticity that permits organisms to mould their form to prevailing circumstances" and (2) "Darwinian. . . selection upon genetic variation." Possibly adaptive behavioral responses include (3) "cultural adaptation (with heritability imposed by learning)" (Waterlow 1985, 1) as well as (4) individual decisions on how to react to stress, strain, or damage. The biology-behavior distinction is really a continuum, because an unknown but substantial proportion of (3) and (4)—including flexibility, adaptive range, and "capacity to develop physiological adaptations" (Waterlow 1985)—is preprogrammed by (2) and perhaps by earlier demonstrations of (1). An illustration is Beaton's (1985) concern that, in humans, phenotypic plasticity in reducing infant growth under energy stress leads to adult shortness that inhibits subsequent adaptations. As suggested earlier, however, similar concerns apply to plasticity that increases tallness, or indeed to lack of plasticity in face of the earlier stress. But the pragmatic distinction between "metabolic and genetic-biological processes" and "socio-behavioral modifications. . .the leading strategy in economizing energy expenditure" made by Ferro-Luzzi (1985, 61) is accepted here. In face of identical and less-than-extreme sequences of threat of undernutrition, genetically and phenotypically identical animals with identical histories can in principle behave differently but cannot differ in biological response. Humans have the unique capacity to think through and plan behavioral responses; for example, to reject the option of working less when under mild energy stress, because that option (even if adaptive) reduces income and therefore prospects for improved well-being later on. Such behavioral planning may involve inadvertently selecting among, compelling, or altering biological responses.
- Whether or not stress (or strain or damage) to an organism is diagnosed depends on what is considered to be its needed or desired functions. For instance, moderate stunting (without wasting) in children diminishes adult capacity for tasks requiring heavy muscular efforts but may increase such capacity in the case of tasks requiring mainly translation of body weight, since there is less need to use effort in moving one's weight about, both during work and while one moves to and from it (see Chapter 5).

3

Time and Stress

Several types of biological and behavioral adjustments to meet current energy stress are distinguished here. The wide range of outcomes, however, reflects the integral effects of different time-patterns of stress, strain, or damage.

There are, as it were, three "clocks" that time the sources, effects, or outcomes of energy stress. The first clock—that of individual birth, growth, aging, procreation, and death—regulates growth and development of individuals and their descendants. A second clock—that of family formation, growth, and separation—is the household cycle, determining when the household is most vulnerable to energy stress. A third, environmental clock—that of changing seasons, climatically varying years, and structurally developing economies—regulates food inflows, prices, and work; for poor rural households, this clock is related mainly to agricultural production. The sequences of source, stress, strain, and damage—and the prospects of adaptation and of its acceptability—depend on the joint action of these three clocks.

Individual Growth and Development

The clock of growth and development measures three time spans through which nutritional stress can affect the ultimate body size of individuals. First, there are individual effects of stress; principally those of inadequate food intake, interacting with illness early in life and influencing growth through adolescence. Second, there are intergenerational changes in body size caused by extended periods of stress. Third, there is the Darwinian mechanism of selection upon genetic variation, which tends to select for shorter body stature in areas where there has been continuous nutritional stress (Tanner 1964). (See the section on intergenerational change in this chapter and that on growth and body size in Chapter 5.)

Individual's Period of Growth and Development

Environmental conditions during the critical period of early childhood affect the size of individuals as adults. In very early life (0-2 years), significant energy stress normally and swiftly reduces the child's growth. The source of such stress is usually inadequate (or reduced) intake of food, or high (or increased) levels of infection or parasites, or both. At this age, a child will respond in a relatively reversible fashion to early short-term stress by following the period of restricted growth with a period of rapid "catch-up" in height.

However, with increasing age, this potential for reversible responses (for effective resistance to energy stress) is progressively reduced. Height growth becomes more and more irreversibly "programmed" onto a lower path, though body weight may be maintained in normal proportion to the reduced height. With the resumption of rapid height growth at adolescence, some capacity for catch-up may be regained (see, for example, the account given in Eveleth 1985, 32). Indian boys severely undernourished in early childhood "achieved greater linear increments [aged 5-20] than well-nourished British or American boys [yet] only 3 cm. of the initial 21 cm. height deficit [was] eliminated" (Ashworth and Millward 1986, 158).

Smaller final adult stature (tolerance of strain) is thus a reflection of the fact that losses of growth in early life are never fully made up. However, the mechanism of growth control shows a degree of plasticity, that is, a capacity—even after initial stress—to respond to future insults, such as infection, by returning to a lower, but parallel, growth curve. This is one of the ways in which the organism responds to information about the outside world: about the levels of disease, food supply, and so forth, current or likely to be encountered in the future. Whether such responses are adaptive or acceptable, that is, the nature and extent of any possible damage, will be discussed later.

Intergenerational Changes in Growth and Size

The effects of tolerance of this environmentally induced energy strain, that is, of smaller body size and growth, can be carried over time spans longer than one generation. Because shorter girls grow up to be shorter women—a fact that is of particular policy importance in the populations where small girls suffer from discrimination in nutrition or health care—they eventually tend to have smaller, slower-growing children. (These populations are mainly in North India and Bangladesh, and not in Sub-Saharan Africa [Harriss 1986; Schofield 1979; Svedberg 1989].) This happens because the amount of food that is taken in by the pregnant woman and transmitted to the fetus, and the space for it to grow in the womb, are both smaller if she is smaller. Hence, even before genetic effects are considered, populations exposed to long periods of stress respond by reducing both growth rates and final adult body size. When the stress is reduced, increases are seen in size, attained at all ages, over one or two generations. Whether such response is adaptive or, if so, acceptable is dealt with in Chapter 5.

Genetic Changes in Body Size

Groups that have lived in the same environment for several generations, and that are largely endogamous, probably select against gene values that impair response to energy stress. Large people are ill-equipped to handle prolonged food shortages. They are also ill-equipped to work in humid heat (Lee 1977), so it cannot be said with certainty that the selection for smallness that appears to exist in many tropical populations is in fact due to energy stress or to the needs of the work environment. Even the very low body mass index (BMI) of some Indian agricultural workers (Shetty 1984), while it too may well be in part genetic, could be traceable to selection of persons for ability to earn livelihoods by hard work in humid heat rather than (or as well as) for better survival prospects under energy stress.

The existence of adaptive, evolutionary adjustments in body size is hinted at by some genetic differences, although relatively minor, in stature between ethnic groups. These can be demonstrated quite early. Well-off (energy-unconstrained) Asian boys have average heights at seven years of age that correspond to the 25th percentile of the National Center for Health Statistics (NCHS) reference growth standard, whereas well-off Africans, Latin Americans, and North Americans of the same age average close to the 50th percentile, that is, about 3.5 centimeters taller (Martorell 1985, 15-16). The Asian height lag is almost certainly genetic, at least in part (Davies 1988). In some populations, the endogenous control mechanism responsible for controlling height can be studied directly. Adult male Pygmies, whose heights average 32 centimeters less than Europeans, have correspondingly lower blood levels of insulin-like growth factor throughout childhood and adolescence (Merimée et al. 1987). It is worth noting that these facts probably reflect adaptive interactions between genetics and environment (Seckler 1985), that is, they are not "ethnic"; for example, mountain populations in many parts of the world, with quite distinct ethnic backgrounds, almost all have small modal adult body size.

Household Life-Cycle Patterns of Stress

A second clock integrates the effects of individual (and to a small extent intergenerational) changes in body size over the members of a household and thus governs the timing of energy stress within its life cycle. Households over the course of their existence have varying ability to meet the (also varying) energy requirements of their members. A household having a high proportion of older children will have a greater capability of providing for its own energy needs than will a household consisting of a large proportion of small children. As children get older, they begin to contribute income to the household so that per capita income increases; this reduces potential energy stress. Then, as the income-earning children leave the home and the aging parents are more likely to be ill, there is again an increased likelihood that the household will experience energy stress. The Malaysian findings of Datta and Meerman (1980) suggest that most rural households experience a cycle of per capita income as follows:

1. Immediately following marriage, both husband and wife tend to earn income; per capita income is quite high, reducing the risk of energy stress.

2. With the arrival of small children, there are more mouths to feed, but no additional income-earners. Indeed, the mother must devote time

to child care, which cuts her income-earning capabilities. The household suffers increased risk of energy stress.

3. As the children grow older, they are able to contribute to income-earning and there are decreased demands on mother's time for child care. Thus there is decreased risk of energy stress.

4. Finally, the income-generating children leave home and parents are at greater risk of being ill, so there is increased risk of energy stress caused by a decline in command over food.

Household income per capita for Malaysia fell as the age of the head of household rose from 25.0 to 37.5 and again from 50.0 to 62.5 years (Datta and Meerman 1980). This was based on cross-sectional data, which frequently lead to ambiguous results. They could indicate that the poor marry later within these intervals; however, there is much evidence that the reverse is true in rural areas of developing countries (Lipton 1983b, 24-27). Much more probably, the results reflect changing economic conditions; but such changes could take place in the economy or in the household. Since not only gross national product (GNP) per person, but also (albeit more slowly) poverty reduction, was advancing in Malaysia over the period, the fall in income as the head of household grew older probably reflected the above household life cycle.[4,5] In western India, evidence from village surveys suggests that life-cycle variation in household income per person is an important source of poverty (low consumption per person) only to the extent that some groups of households, experiencing such variation, are for reasons of ascription (such as caste) very unlikely to obtain land or high-earning jobs. Such people cannot readily borrow in years of hardship because they do not appear to potential lenders to be certain to repay (Lipton 1983c, 55-57).

How important is this family cycle for undernutrition and possible adaptation to it? Obviously, the household tends to be at higher risk of energy stress just when the children's early growth and development are taking place. In severely income-constrained environments, there is therefore likely to be stunting due to energy stress. However, children may be able to contribute at an early age to household income so that energy stress is reduced and—provided that their energy expenditure at work is moderate and that, as the evidence suggests (Schofield 1979), an adequate proportion of extra household income is devoted to calories for youngsters—they enjoy catch-up growth. Genetic capacity to defer the growth spurt (latency) is likely to be selected for if child labor is

---

[4]Panel data are needed before confident assertions can be made about the household's energy stress cycle—or even its income cycle. However, it is clear that the extended or joint family (Lipton 1983c) does not present a pervasive exception to this cycle in less-developed countries. Nor does polygamy, which (apart from requiring unusually wealthy men) implies, if pervasive, highly skewed sex ratios, much earlier marriage for men than for women (and frequent separations), or a large proportion of single adult men—phenomena that are not at all common.

[5]Furthermore, income per person is a less satisfactory indicator of household well-being than expenditure per adult-equivalent. Nevertheless the data of Datta and Meerman (1980) are suggestive: the evidence for a household-cycle relationship in Malaysia is further examined in Lipton 1983c.

resorted to for many generations, and if, but only if, short height in adulthood does not, up to the completion of the couple's normal period of reproduction, confer offsetting reductions in fitness.

Such child labor, however, may involve unacceptable costs of school time. If primary education were universal, and if its providers (far from seeking to recover its costs) were also to compensate poor rural parents for the lost income from child labor, this consequence would be avoided. Whether either government or local communities of very poor countries could afford to do this, however, is not clear.

Since these sequences of the household cycle (like seasonal fluctuations) are obvious to couples from long experience, why cannot households anticipate them and smooth out levels of food intake per adult-equivalent (avoidance of source of stress)? If households' future earnings prospects are very low or uncertain, they may not be able to avoid seasonal or life-cycle energy stress by borrowing to cover added expenditures required when household food needs are high relative to household current resources. Also, very poor households may be unable to store grain (or cash) against expected high energy demands in late pregnancy or lactation. Finally, such households presumably lack access to either traditional or modern social security. Unfortunately, it is exactly the most vulnerable (poor) groups who are likely to face these problems, together with credit-market imperfections due to the need to spread the fixed cost of loan administration for small borrowers over a small loan—unless given by someone with special local knowledge, who is likely to be a powerful person in local credit markets and to have few if any local competitors.

The small role of formal social security shifts attention to extended kin networks, long-term employer responsibilities, or other aspects of cohesion of the social structure as possible means of assisting adaptation to periods of stress in the household cycle. Such cohesion has been noted by many anthropologists as a major safety measure against another source of energy stress: drought-induced hunger and disorder. In Yaavahalli village in South India, during a severe drought in the mid-1960s, the lack of deaths directly resulting from the lack of food has been attributed to the way in which the population organized the collective flow of human energy. According to the local people, the main indigenous mechanism for keeping famine at bay was the preservation of the large family unit. Anthropological observation confirmed that larger households achieved economies of scale in well-being per unit of consumption (compare Lazear and Michael 1980 for U.S. data), apart from raising consumption per adult-equivalent by smoothing out family cycle effects (Maclachlan 1983, 3).

Apart from avoiding the source of stress by the choice of long-term size or structure of family and household, some families split or combine when the stress occurs, thus repartitioning the stress to prevent severe strain. This response of altering the household cycle to improve security when drought or famine threatens a risky period for energy stress merits closer attention in response to Ferro-Luzzi's (1985, 61) plea to remedy the paucity of information on such methods of "energy-sparing" behavioral adaptation. In Yaavahalli, the elders defined their tasks as "securing social harmony" during the drought so as to prevent the fragmentation of families at a time when smaller households would be most vulnerable to the adverse conditions: families were ordered to abstain from discussing controversial subjects that might lead to arguments. "The prevention of social disruption was thus a prominent feature of their famine management strategies" (Maclachlan 1983, 228). Energy and food were conserved through the cancellation of nonessential Hindu ceremonies and the eating of food on alternate days. Wealthier village members helped poorer members by giving gifts. In other South Indian villages, where social bonding had been eroded through migration and a closer integration with the cash economy, hunger-related deaths were frequent (Maclachlan 1983, 273). The nutritional adequacy of Yaavahalli, in face of family cycles superimposed on drought stress, was intricately bound to the maintenance of respect for stable, if static, social obligations.

Economists have found some evidence of economies of scale in consumption for the household (Lazear and Michael 1980; Deaton, Ruiz-Castillo, and Thomas 1984). However, these studies were made among not-so-poor households. There are likely to be fewer economies of scale in energy consumption among the very poor, probably those relating only to cooking and storage of food. But even small economies are crucial under stress, especially if acceptable adaptation means sustaining body size or growth above some critical point (see discussion in Chapter 5 under "Risk of Death"). In particular, if fuelwood is in short supply, perhaps because of the increasing cost of energy expenditure for its collection, then economies of scale could be very important.

Furthermore, Indian household surveys strongly suggest that large families suffer somewhat smaller downward fluctuation in income because they (1) often comprise parents and married children, and in technologically stagnant agriculture, where most poverty is concentrated, past experience by the parents of coping with climatically bad seasons is significant in reducing losses of farm income (Rosenzweig and Wolpin 1985); and (2) have better chances that some members will migrate to places where incomes are not strongly covariant with those of the home village, so that remaining family residents enjoy much better expectations of income transfer when their own (village-based) incomes fluctuate downward (Rosenzweig 1988). However, these accounts, while providing rigorous quantitative evidence of such "economies to family size in consumption-risk reduction" (as one may call them), also show that the effects are small—and considerably smaller still for those with few land assets, who are likeliest to be poorest and hence at most nutritional risk from fluctuations.

Time-Patterns of Environmental Stress

There are two patterns of stress for which timing depends on the environment. First, within a year, there are seasonal variations in the scarcity (and hence often the price) of food, the intensity and duration of labor, and the incidence of infection; especially if covariant, these will increase the risk of stress at certain times. Second, year-on-year variability of crop yields can result in extreme stress in famine years.

Seasonal Timing of Stress

The seasonal nature of production of food, especially in one-season agricultures, means that peak seasons for energy expenditure—notably the late wet season—often arrive when food stores are depleted and prices high. Thus peak availability and peak expenditure of energy often do not coincide. Transport costs, labor movement or information costs, or the costs and difficulties in storage or borrowing sometimes prevent poor households from readily transferring food or work over space or over time. The problem is worst when the exact timing of seasonal stress is hard to predict, when it is compounded by a bad previous harvest (and thus unusually small food stores or cash savings), or when it overlaps with personal stress, especially from illness (often itself seasonal).

Such seasonal stress, when it happens, tends to hit most rural households in an area together. The usual repartitioning devices (see previous section), and also borrowing and storage, are therefore less readily available. Seasonal stress can be found even where there are two or three crops a year (for example, in Bangladesh [Clay 1981]), or where there is little climatic seasonality (for example, in Papua New Guinea [Crittenden and Baines 1986]). The type of energy stress, that is, reduced intakes or increased expenditure, is important for identifying the nature of appropriate policy initiatives. In addition, the point at which functional impairment occurs, within what may be a relatively short period of stress, is similarly important. Studies on seasonality and nutrition have been reviewed by Longhurst and Payne (1981), and Teokul, Payne, and Dugdale (1986). Annegers (1973) shows that in West Africa the classical seasonal pattern of energy deficit (the hungry season) occurred in about 7 out of 10 cases. Where it did not, intake rose to meet increased energy expenditure.

Although an area such as the highlands of Papua New Guinea is aseasonal with regard to rainfall, there is seasonality in the labor demands of the two agricultural subsystems: mixed gardens and sweet-potato fields. Seasonal patterns of births and mixed garden activity are linked ritually (Crittenden and Baines 1986). This is probably so as to avoid the seasonal coincidence of heavy family work and scarce food together with children reaching the age of 6-12 months, at which age they are in between the phases of passive and active immunity, and hence especially vulnerable to infections (Schofield 1974). The consequences of failure thus to avoid the source of stress are well described by McGregor et al. (1968, especially p. 343) with regard to marked seasonal impacts on growth of children aged under two years in The Gambia. In communities that do avoid unfavorable birth timing, "catch-up attention" leads to the correction of quite substantial seasonal fluctuations in mean birthweight (150- to 450-gram differences are reported from several countries). By six to seven months of age in a New Guinea sample (Ferro-Luzzi, Pastore, and Sette 1988), these differences were no longer detectable. This seasonal adjustment of childbearing is also very clearly seen in Bangladesh.

As suggested above, cycles of energy intake and expenditure (through food and work) are sometimes linked to cycles of conception and birth, the latter peaking after harvest time (Dyson and Crook 1981).

Seasonal maternal activities (such as farm work) that reduce breastfeeding frequency contribute to this seasonal pattern (Schofield 1979; Quandt 1984). Several studies have shown how pregnant women can lose weight through the wet season at this time (Rowland et al. 1981; Pagezy 1984), but recent evidence on adaptation in pregnancy (reviewed in Chapter 4) suggests that this is less risky to the women's health than was once believed.

Direct effects of climatic stress on human fertility may also influence seasonal patterns of birthrates (Mosher 1979). Increases in prolactin, which would somewhat inhibit fertility, have been associated with energy stress, and Huffman (1983) has suggested that the increase in prolactin from dry to wet season could be due to such effects rather than to decreases in calorie intakes or body weight as such. If so, this biological resistance to strain (in seasonal agricultures) prevents both further strain on the mother via first-trimester pregnancy in the wet season and high risk to the child via underfeeding in the fetus throughout the wet season.

Seasonal changes in energy stress have a differential impact within the family, a point explored more fully in Chapter 7 under "Age and Sex Groups." The conventional wisdom is that in times of food scarcity the impact falls more heavily on women and children. However, this has not been found in one recent study (Abdullah and Wheeler 1985). Even if it were the case, it might be adaptive, because women appear better able to tolerate damage from strains due to seasonal stress if all else fails, and in general to survive energy stress better than men, according to recent research in Senegal (Rosetta 1986), a point further explored in Chapter 5 under "Changes in Specific Metabolic Rates of Tissues: Metabolic Adaptation."

The balance of biological and economic reasoning suggests that most people have adapted to normal seasonal stress. Biology would suggest that, since such stress is a regular occurrence, it comes to involve a cycle of body-reserve depletion and repletion, and to reflect "trade-offs, between the advantages of reduced food storage losses on the one hand and [of] year-round constancy of body weight on the other" (Dugdale and Payne 1987, 241). Anticipation, leading to storage, borrowing, and so forth (to an extent limited by the costs of such precautions) might be expected to occur in the face of regular and hence predictable seasonal variation in energy intake and outgo if such variation cannot be adequately "looked after" by biological adjustments. However, problems would arise when the timing or effect of the lean season is uncertain; when methods of handling it are disrupted by market failure, by worsening income distribution, and so forth; or when a bad season is compounded by an illness or by the carryover effects of a previous bad year.

Bad Years and Stress

There is considerable interannual variation in energy intake caused by the uncertainty of food production, both directly (for subsistence farmers) and via dearer food (for poorer laborers, townspeople, and food-deficit, including many cash crop, farmers). The consequences of this variability are more serious if the stress is prolonged or repeated. Many rural communities expect interannual variations (for example, "famine one year in seven"); obviously, the reserves available to cope will be more easily exhausted with a prolonged period of stress. Thus, higher levels of functional impairment (morbidity, mortality) would be expected as a result of these extended stresses, though the empirical data are weak (Longhurst 1986).

Families and individuals undergo a sequence of responses when faced with annual nutritional stresses (Jodha 1975; Dirks 1980; Campbell and Trechter 1982; Watts 1983; Longhurst 1986). The Jodha-Watts-Longhurst formulation of progressively more serious adjustments during a cycle from breakdown back to full recovery is as follows:

1. The first is domestic mutual support—identification of "fallback" activities of household members, including gathering of foods, and restructuring of current farm activities to maximize effective availability of products, including a variety of salvage operations. This is, in essence, avoidance of much of the source of stress.

2. The second response is another avoidance of the source of stress—minimization of current commitments through suspension or cancellation of normal obligations, including deferral or default on grain loans and tax.

3. The source of stress cannot be avoided in many cases but can be repartitioned across households or over time by consumption, or sale in exchange for cheaper energy sources, of inventories of home-produced foods or purchased foods—at the expense of intended uses such as marriage, village charitable relief, sale when prices rise, or acquisition of client's or patron's support.

4. The next stage also involves repartitioning of the source over time, via sale or mortgage of assets, with a sequence based on liquidity and productivity of assets and with a preference toward mortgage rather than sale.

5. Next is short- or long-term migration (repartitioning of stress within the household).

6. Only after some strain has been resisted or tolerated do households usually take up access to the stress avoidance strategy of famine relief from state or patron assistance; this strategy may permit reversal of the earlier costlier strategies, for example, by return, recovery, replanting, and reconstitution of reserves.

Households, individuals, and communities where this sequence of responses has broken down will be subject to strain. Jodha (1975) emphasizes that most households sampled by him during successive bad seasons accepted reductions in energy intake, even to possibly dangerous levels, before seeking to dispose of, or even to mortgage, productive assets.

4

Sources and Types of Stress

Energy is available to the body from the oxidation of food and is expended as heat and work. Any factor increasing energy expenditure at a given level of intake (or maintaining it at, in some sense, a "high" level relative to intake) is a source of energy stress. So, for a given rate of energy expenditure, is any factor reducing (or keeping "low") energy intake or its conversion efficiency into heat or work. Energy stress has undesirable effects on anthropometry only if it causes adult body mass or child growth to fall to levels that threaten functions or capabilities, that is, to fall below the acceptable range. Hence this report emphasizes the impact of various types of stress on vulnerable groups, to whose members it is likely to cause strain and perhaps damage (the poor, preschoolers, and so forth), rather than on, say, obese adults, for whom energy stress (reduced diet, increased exercise) is often medically recommended.

However, particular types of stress may cause strain, via nonanthropometric effects that are undesirable in themselves, even on persons not already small. Sudden extreme effort can damage the untrained heart; reduced intake even of an initially balanced diet (for example, in response to reduced expenditure) can result in micronutrient deficiencies (Buzina et al. 1989); infections and parasites are obviously bad ways to lose weight. And all three sorts of events, even when risk-free, are unpleasant.

Reduced Energy Inputs

Food Consumption

Obviously, anything leading to a reduction of an initially just-adequate level of food consumption, unmatched by sufficiently reduced energy expenditure or increased metabolic efficiency or both, is a source of stress that is likely to produce strain. The most common reason is a decline in the food entitlement of the household, that is, in its claims upon food, either in the marketplace or from domestic, customary, or legally mandated (for example, employer's meals, social security) sources. Such a decline may result from crop failure, loss of employment income, seasonal rises in food prices, or an interannual combination of food and income shortages, as in conditions of famine. At the level of the individual, consumption may be reduced because of voluntary or forced changes in intrahousehold allocation of food, or very commonly because of loss of appetite following an infection or other disease episode. For example, studies of such episodes in Bangladesh have shown up to 40 percent reduction in energy intake of small children, which could not be overcome by encouragement to eat more (Hoyle, Yunus, and Chen 1980).

Appetite can also be reduced because of a decline in the quality of food available. The diets of poor people, particularly in rural settings, are often monotonously dependent upon one or two staple sources of energy. This can result in marginal levels of intake of micronutrients—vitamins, minerals, essential fatty acids—lack of which, besides possibly reducing the efficiency of metabolism of dietary energy, may also reduce appetite (Miller 1982).

Finally, the transition from breast milk to solid foods constitutes one of the periods of greatest potential energy stress. Many cereal-based, and especially root-based, gruels or porridges are either so thick as to be difficult for small children to masticate (so that feeding requires lengthy and intensive supervision) or so much thinned by adding water as to have a low energy content per unit of volume when cooked. In either case, young infants may have difficulty in consuming sufficient volumes of food to maintain the growth (sustained positive energy balance) that they achieved when feeding on the breast. Wandel and Holmboe-Ottesen (1992) describe how these sources of stress—almost always leading to strain—are exacerbated when small children accompany mothers to work in the fields. If an infection or other trauma occurs during this period, the combination of low energy density and loss of appetite may result in a high level of energy stress—especially as the normal weaning period of 6-12 months is typically one when (for many infections) passive immunity has been lost but active immunity not yet fully acquired.

Food Energy Retention

After food has been consumed, the next step in the process of energy conversion is absorption. The accepted normal coefficients of digestibility of the energy substrates in foods are high (usually more than 90 percent of the available energy content of foodstuffs is absorbed). During illness, however, absorption can be reduced. Earlier studies (Chung and Viscorova 1948) suggested that gastrointestinal infections may be sources of energy stress by causing substantial reduction of absorption rates. More recent studies (Molla et al. 1983) indicated that the magnitude may be relatively small and dependent on the specific types of pathogens involved: watery diarrheas, for example, seem to result in quite small reductions in the efficiency of absorption.

There are, of course, other mechanisms by which these and other infections act as sources of stress. They induce lower energy intake through anorexia, and they lead to increased energy requirements to fuel biological resistance to infection, as indicated by higher-than-normal body temperature.

A recent study of the three main forms of schistosomiasis assesses its effect in reducing not only food intake (via anorexia) but also food energy retention. The parasites affect each of the three sequential requirements for food energy use: absorption through the gastrointestinal tract, utilization of nutrients absorbed, and retention (nonexcretion) of partly utilized nutrients (Stephenson 1987a, 2-3). Between ages 6 and 16 months, treatment with metrifonate of children with nonsevere *S. hematobium* (some also had hookworm) resulted in a 50 percent (0.8 kilogram) increase in weight gain, compared with children given a placebo, during the six months subsequent to treatment. "Metrifonate treatment of even light and moderate infections . . . results in a much greater improvement in general health status of children than was previously thought" (Stephenson 1987b, 59-60), probably because some or all of the three components of food energy use (here called "food energy retention") have been substantially improved. This implies that such parasites—perhaps more than most infections, and despite the fact that their own consumption (unlike that of some other gut worms) is negligible—substantially affect "extended absorption" and hence energy stress.

Raised Expenditure

Physical Activity

Maintenance metabolism normally accounts for 50-75 percent of energy requirements. However, it is less adjustable than energy expenditure on physical activity—the most obvious and perhaps the most important variable component on the output side of the balance sheet. Recent work suggests that energy expenditure among Scottish women is below the basal metabolic rate (BMR) of 1.4 (Nestlé Foundation 1987), but in poor laboring communities, especially in busy seasons, higher rates would be expected. Thus, an adult man may increase his daily expenditure rate by more than 40 percent during periods of heavy work preparing land for planting (Bleiburg, Brun, and Goiham 1980). Also, when individuals previously adapted to a more sedentary regime undertake prolonged hard physical work (not just distance running [Miller 1982] but also presumably the seasonal clearing of heavy bush or weeding rice), resting metabolic rates (RMRs) rise above their normal level for 15-24 hours afterward. This work-induced thermogenesis combines with (Miller would say it potentiates) the thermogenesis that follows eating meals—the so-called diet-induced thermogenesis (see Chapter 5). Although relatively small (less than 5 percent of total expenditure), this combined effect could significantly increase the size of an energy stress originating from increased workload in the absence of an equivalent rise in food intake.

Pregnancy

The deposition of energy during pregnancy seems obviously to imply increased overall needs. Thus, the cost of laying down new tissue in the fetus, placenta, and mammary glands can be calculated on theoretical grounds to be around 40,000 kilocalories. It might be expected that these additions to total body weight would also give rise to an increase in basal metabolism on a pro rata basis, above the nonpregnant level. This would suggest a further 30,000 kilocalories distributed over the course of pregnancy (Hytten and Leitch 1971). In practice, however, many surveys in both industrial and developing-country populations (Durnin 1988) have shown little or no increase in food energy intake until the last few weeks of pregnancy, and even then by much smaller amounts than these calculations would suggest. It seems that compensatory downward adjustments in BMR, in some cases together with reductions in physical activity, can be sufficient to almost neutralize the energy stress of pregnancy. For example, in The Gambia, measured reductions in BMR were such as to imply a net increase in total requirements of only 1,000 kilocalories over the entire pregnancy (Dunn Nutrition Unit 1986, 30). Maintenance energy metabolism adjusts throughout pregnancy, declining by about 10 percent during the first two trimesters and rising above the normal level only during the last. As a result, Durnin et al. (1985) have concluded that there is no need to increase energy intake during pregnancy unless there is a significant increase in physical activity by the pregnant woman.

Seriously reduced birthweight undeniably increases the baby's risks of early death (and of lesser degrees of damage), and some constellations of energy intake, energy expenditure, and metabolic rates in pregnancy can seriously reduce birthweight. However, it also seems that pregnant women's capacity to reduce BMR normally prevents these constellations, even in poor rural households, except in extreme situations of reduced intake (especially in the third trimester), or if energy expenditure is too high. In such cases, for example, in The Gambia, "dietary supplementation . . . increase[d] birthweight . . . [yet without] effect . . . on weight . . . gain during pregnancy," but a repartitioning of source of stress appears to be available: apparently, more maternal meals (not calories) per day "increased the number of post-prandial glucose peaks [with] beneficial effect on fetal growth" (Lawrence, McKillop, and Durnin 1989, 72).

Recent work funded by the Nestlé Foundation (1987) has found that—although initially often small and lean—rural women in three less-developed countries benefit, with regard to their prospects of producing a healthy child, from nutrition supplements in pregnancy only if the second or third trimester occurs during the wet season. A study in Thailand in the Nestlé program illustrates the converse: that "pregnant women who had the second half of their pregnancy [in] the dry season worked significantly harder and had smaller babies" (Mo-Suwan 1989, 601). In other words, what matters for small mothers, who do not have the option of increasing energy intake, is to avoid heavy fieldwork: "rest is best" (Briend 1984). Only with this form of avoidance of source of stress can women be confident of producing a healthy child with little or no increase in energy intake during pregnancy (Mo-Suwan 1989). However, this depends upon factors operating in combination with the metabolic responses described above.

Many at-risk women (though the proportion depends upon traditional customs and conventions) are normally involved in productive work and in social exchanges. By curtailing these, women can achieve significant reductions in energy expenditure over the whole period, as compared with the nonpregnant state (Durnin 1988; McNeill and Payne 1985). In addition, the work reported by Dunn Nutrition Unit (1986,

30-31) and Nestlé (1987) is finding that metabolic "adaptations" to reduce energy stress in pregnancy are greatest where (as in The Gambia) unsupplemented women are normally exposed to considerable energy stress. They resist strain by more efficient metabolic conversion—and do this most when stress (within tolerable limits) is greatest" (Dunn Nutrition Unit 1986, 31). This work on pregnant women provides possibly the most striking example to date of adaptive changes in metabolic efficiency. In pregnancy at least, it seems that mechanisms of resistance to strain exist that increase efficiency (at least if the stress of pregnancy is not accompanied by extra stress from heavy physical work), and that these mechanisms are of sufficient magnitude to permit without visible strain a fully successful outcome even with relatively small increases in intake.

Lactation

Lactation increases expenditure progressively through the period of suckling, with final rates of up to 1,000 kilocalories per day for the energy content of milk, plus the energy cost of production. Efficiency of milk production has been found to be about 80 percent (Thomson, Hytten, and Billewicz 1970). However, recent research suggests that lactating women on low energy intakes continue to have low BMRs, at least to the same degree as in pregnancy, which would reduce net lactation stress from 1,000 kilocalories per day to, say, 850-900 kilocalories per day. Lawrence found that "in Gambian women maternal BMR values drop to some 10 percent below nonpregnant, nonlactating values following parturition and remain there throughout the whole of the first year of lactation" (Dunn Nutrition Unit 1986). During this time, indeed, "BMR was reduced by up to 100 kcals/day [even] compared with conception and late lactation," although very little fat loss, and (except in the first month of lactation) no reduction in physical activity, was observed (Lawrence and Whitehead 1989, 179). These results were not replicated (Prentice and Prentice 1988) for well-fed Cambridge mothers. This again suggests—this time for lactation—that metabolic adaptation to resist moderate strain in the reproductive cycle is available in proportion to need. However, testing of the Gambian findings on lactation over a range of different environments and ethnic backgrounds (as has been achieved in pregnancy studies) is clearly necessary.

Infections and Parasites

Besides effects on absorption, infectious diseases can result in increased expenditure of energy through the effects of enterotoxins. These raise metabolic rate, body temperature, and hence heat losses. Each degree of fever can increase metabolic rate by as much as 8 percent (Briscoe 1979). As discussed earlier in this chapter, the effect of illness upon food energy retention (as on appetite) generally sharpens the impact of these sources of energy stress, in marked contrast to the partly self-correcting adjustments in the case of pregnancy and lactation. The only truly costless adjustment to energy stress in illness is recovery.

Altitude

High (or increased) altitude increases the physiological stress of a given amount of work because of the reduced pressure of oxygen. This results in many physiological responses, including metabolic changes. Hypoxia and malnutrition commonly coexist, for example, in the Andes, where most research has been carried out. Studies summarized in Haas 1983 show that the effects of altitude on fetal, infant, and child growth are compounded with those of undernutrition. In these populations hypoxia, cold, undernutrition, and disease are all associated with altitude; all combine to challenge nutritional status and are plainly unpleasant. However, there seems to be an adaptive resistance to strain. Infants at high altitudes develop a large chest early in growth, resulting in a slightly greater weight (for relatively somewhat shorter stature) than in equally healthy low-altitude children. Haas's (1983, 51) warning against inferring that a large chest is adaptive at high altitude appears to be unduly cautious. The benefits of this may well show in other respects, through age-related changes in heart function, blood pressure, and so forth.

For adults' work, as well as children's play, energy requirements are increased by changing altitude (gradient, hilliness) as well as by high altitude. Moreover, "the same increase in grade will increase energy expenditure by a greater amount [for successive increments in] speed, grade, or load, or a combination of these"—and the downs do not compensate for the ups. "The energy cost of walking downhill on a –10 percent grade . . . was higher than the cost of walking at approximately the same speed and load . . . on the level" (Pimental and Pandolf 1979).

Studies from Papua New Guinea (Crittenden and Baines 1985; Bogen and Crittenden 1987) have explored whether altitude can provide an index of the degree of stress created by an environment—an index that can be correlated with indicators of malnutrition. As in Haas's (1983) analysis, there are too many factors involved for the effect of altitude on energy stress to be isolated. Activity patterns may be different—that is, more walking (Ohtsuka et al. 1985)—for reasons only partly linked to altitude. Certainly, lowland children were taller than children in intermediate and higher zones. However, altitude per se (in Papua New Guinea), except where it limits economic opportunity, was not a sufficient explanation for malnutrition. It is clear, however, that a group adapted to lowland life that migrates to a much higher altitude (and therefore increases the cost of oxygen acquisition per unit of work done) must respond to this potential source of energy stress in some way, either by repartitioning expenditure patterns in the direction of more productive work in order to secure increased intakes, or by tolerating a change in body size.

Temperature

There is a range of temperature, the so-called thermoneutral range (about 25-38°C for a naked man), over which the core temperature of the body is maintained constant by means of physiological mechanisms rather than metabolic responses. Within this range, heat losses are regulated by controlling heat transfer from core to exterior, and hence skin temperature. Metabolic thermoregulation occurs whenever cold or heat stress from the environment threatens to bring a person outside the limits of thermal neutrality. Rises in VO_2 and in metabolic rate, in response to such stresses, have long been established in newborn infants (Schulze 1986, 29).

The two mechanisms involved in thermogenesis, that is, in the production of heat above the thermoneutral level in response to cold stress,[6] are shivering (the conversion of chemical energy to mechanical work inside the body) and nonshivering (the direct oxidation of energy stores through increased metabolism in tissues, such as brown fat, to produce heat) (see, for example, Rothwell and Stock 1979). Similarly, elevated heat loss can be achieved in response to heat stress, that is, at temperatures above thermal neutrality, by increased evaporative losses from the lungs or from the skin as sweat, or both. These processes will themselves require additional energy because of the osmotic work involved in the excretion of sweat. This will ultimately have to be derived from the diet, just as a heater or a refrigerator needs a power source. Some experimental studies have claimed to demonstrate an increase in requirements due to heat stress on top of heavy work loads. In theory, therefore, the energy requirements for sustaining a given work load might be increased by cold stress[7] or by heat stress. However, there are complications to this simple model of a fixed thermoneutral range of outside temperatures, with biological mechanisms of control coming into play at the upper and lower ends in order to stabilize body temperatures.

First of all, the location of the lower range of outside temperatures depends upon behavior: the naked ape puts on clothes and hence reduces loss of heat from the skin. At lower temperatures he retreats into a house; lower still, and he lights a fire (if he can afford the fuel). All these strategies, by raising the temperature of the immediate living environment, lower the outside temperature at which shivering or metabolic thermogenesis occurs. Failure to do so causes great discomfort. Thus avoidance of source of stress is the first response to cold.

In rare cases, resistance has been observed. The !Kung Bushmen are able to reduce their core temperature and hence RMR so as to retain lower skin temperatures and hence lower heat losses than other ethnic groups. Both avoidance and resistance strategies mean that some cold stress can be handled—apparently at very low cost—without extra thermogenesis, energy intake, or reduced activity.

---

[6]Other triggers of thermogenesis are dealt with in Chapter 5 under "Adjustment of Thermogenesis." Some thermogenesis is "diet-induced" and may or may not be (1) functional, (2) reduced, perhaps adaptively, during energy stress. The discussion here is confined to cold stress.

[7]The qualification here is that the metabolic efficiency of muscular work is relatively low (about 30 percent). Depending upon the initial and final circumstances, therefore, it may happen that the "waste heat" generated by physical activity is still sufficient to maintain body temperature without recourse to additional thermogenesis.

The upper limit of thermoneutrality can also change. Acclimatization to high temperatures follows a sequence: first, an increase in sensible (visible) sweat production; later, a more efficient, that is, less energy-expensive, insensible (invisible) loss of water vapor. Petrasek (1978) demonstrated a slight reduction of expenditure and intake by people fully acclimatized to tropical heat.

This complex and somewhat uncertain picture is reflected in the attitude of FAO/WHO committees on energy requirements. The 1950 and 1957 committees recommended a 5 percent decrease in the intake of energy for each 10°C rise in average annual outside dry-bulb temperatures above 10°C. After 1973 no allowance was made, on the dubious grounds that, although there was clearly some rise, its size was reduced by clothing, heating, housing, and indoor work, and that the previous 5 percent figure was too arbitrary to retain (FAO/WHO 1973, 27-28). Work in Japan and Papua New Guinea (Suzuki 1959; Hipsley 1969, 8) strongly confirms the extra energy cost of work when there are quite moderate levels of cold. Except for extreme heat (above, say, 35°C) or unacclimatized subjects, this has not been so clearly shown at the other end of the temperature spectrum. There is, however, quite persuasive evidence (Quenouille et al. 1951; Mason, Jacob, and Balakrishnan 1964) that after making allowances for differences in body size, basal metabolic rates are lower by some 8 percent in warm as opposed to temperate climates, and that individuals moving from one to the other show adaptive changes of this magnitude over a period of a few weeks.

Reduced Conversion Efficiency

The thermodynamic efficiency with which food energy is converted to useful products such as body tissues (including energy stores), milk, and physical work, as distinct from heat, can also vary. As will be seen later, in the section on metabolic adjustments, the extent to which this happens generally, as a compensatory or adaptive adjustment comprising resistance to stress, is controversial. As distinct from this, reduced conversion efficiency could be a source of stress.

There is good evidence that deficient intakes of the B vitamins, and of essential fatty acids, result in a lowering of conversion efficiency of energy into work, with greater heat production and less useful product (Miller 1982). A similar effect may perhaps explain the synergism between anemia and protein-energy malnutrition (Cornu, Pondi Njiki, and Agbor Egbe 1985), and possibly some part of the role of zinc in nutrition.

It is also to be expected that there will be genetic selection for, and conversely sometimes the loss of, characteristics needed for efficient conversion of main staples. This avoidance of source of stress might take place over many generations, as an inherited rejection of individuals with genes conferring energy stress in the presence of specific staples. For instance, groups that have long been transhumants are not likely to contain many individuals whose gene set inhibits them from metabolizing lactose. If this is a general phenomenon, migration—or radical changes in a main food staple—could produce serious energy stress in significant proportions of affected persons.

5

Biological Responses to the Stress Environment

Adjustments to the work process form a bridge between the biological and behavioral responses to the stress environment. Energy stress leads to changes in bodily variables such as height, weight, and the proportion of fat and lean tissues. These changes help to induce both an altered biology *of* work (physical working capacity) and behavioral modifications *at* work (duration, selection of tasks, and performance). The biological responses are considered here; behavioral responses will be discussed in Chapter 6.

At each stage, four questions are addressed. Is the response an avoidance, repartitioning, resistance, or tolerance of the challenge? Is the challenge the source of stress, the stress itself, the strain, or the damage? Is the response adaptive or nonadaptive, given the stress, that is, likely to increase the prospects of survival through the period of producing viable offspring? If the response is adaptive, to what extent is it acceptable, that is, (more or less) fully preservative of capabilities (health and function), with little and brief cost or pain?

There are six types of biological adjustment by which human organisms adapt, acceptably or not, to energy stress, strain, or damage. Most of the responses can take place across any of their personal or environmental time scales, from a single crop season to long-run genetic inheritance, as discussed in Chapter 4.

The first is reduction in body size or growth rate. This is a form of resistance to strain, although, if the stress takes the form of illness, such reduction is perhaps better seen as a resistance to damage. The reduction can be adaptive, that is, fitness-restoring within the changed environment, unless of course it impairs prospects of survival or reproduction. The adaptation can be judged acceptable only if physical and mental capacity, and resistance to disease, are not impaired to the extent that social competence or the quality of life of individuals is reduced.

The second biological adjustment seeks to preempt the risk of strain by repartitioning the stress via a rise in the proportion of body weight comprising tissues or organs of low metabolic activity per kilogram. In increasing order of basal metabolic rate (BMR) per kilogram, the main tissues are bone; fat; nonheart muscles; heart; gut, liver, spleen, and so forth; and brain. Clearly, some such rise in the proportion of low BMR per kilogram tissues could be an effective repartitioning response to energy stress as such; but it could induce other strains and would not be genuine adaptation to the new environment as a whole if these strains tended to disproportionately reduce or destroy survival chances in other respects. Even non-life-threatening adaptations in body composition might be unacceptable (for example, reductions in the brain's share of body mass), while others might not (for example, reductions in a fat share initially above 10-15 percent).

The third and fourth types of adjustment are attempts to resist strain. The third is metabolic adaptation, that is, reduction in specific metabolic activity (metabolic rate per unit mass of one or more tissues or organs). The fourth is increasing overall thermodynamic efficiency by improving the proportion of dietary energy that is converted into useful forms of energy or products; for example, by reducing thermogenesis.

The fifth is involuntary (biologically forced) reduction in the level of physical activity above the resting metabolic rate (RMR); for example, as earlier glycogen exhaustion (following lower energy intake) reduces the proportion of VO_2max at which, for a given period (say, an hour), the body can function. (VO_2max is a measure of the maximum rate of oxidation attainable by an individual in the short term.) Some of these issues of involuntary reduction in work activity are considered below. Others are considered jointly with behavioral responses to energy stress affecting physical activity. These adjustments are forms of tolerance of strain amounting, in some cases, to tolerance of damage.

The sixth adjustment is that of involuntary responses affecting the reproductive cycle. In many situations, these six tend to occur in combinations as "integrated responses," although there may be a hierarchic sequence through which they would come into play under increasing degrees of stress.

Growth and Body Size

This discussion refers to the "acceptability", or otherwise, of adjustments to energy stress (in growth or in body size) that are sustained for at least a year, and in some cases carried through life. Seasonal changes in adult weight normally "appear to be rather modest, rarely exceeding 5 percent of the maximum yearly value of body weight [with questionable] impact on work capacity, on functional competence, and on [adults'] power to initiate adaptive responses" (Ferro-Luzzi, James, and Waterlow 1988, 44). For children (and for birth weights) seasonal fluctuations are more serious, but "factors other than primary energy imbalances," notably illnesses, appear to be the main cause (Ferro-Luzzi, Pastore, and Sette, 1988, 37).

Smallness as a Direct Contribution
to Energy-Saving

Under energy stress, body mass usually decreases, or in the case of growing children, increases more slowly. Does such a response to current energy stress—reducing the weight-for-height or the rate of gain of height or both—result not only in a reduction of current energy needs but also the avoidance of future energy stress? Beaton (1989) points out that the immediate energy saving, involved in reduced growth rates in childhood, is normally in a range of only 2-3 percent of total daily requirements. He draws two conclusions. First, such responses are too small to be a very important component of adaptive strategy. Second, changes in energy supply of this magnitude could not be "sensed" by the individual organism above the level of random fluctuations in both food intake and energy demands; hence the resulting growth adaptations could not be an adaptive response, because they would not be triggered either by the stress itself or by the resulting strain.

Nonetheless, it would seem that the energy saving due to early growth reduction—and the ensuing small adult size—is an important and often adaptive form of resistance to strain, and hence part of the overall strategy of adaptive responses. To recognize how this works, it is necessary to look at energy-saving over a longer period than the single day that Beaton (1989) examines. There is a compound-interest effect. As a child advances along a slower growth curve, so its cumulative energy saving increases rapidly relative to what would have been required for advance along a curve of faster growth.

This is illustrated in Table 2, which compares the energy requirements of a girl whose weight growth is along the 50th percentile of the current U.S. National Center for Health Statistics (NCHS) reference growth standard and those of a girl subject to early growth-faltering. The upper half of the table gives the energy cost per day of BMR, physical activity, and growth, together with the total daily requirement and the cumulative lifetime energy needs for supporting growth along the 50th percentile. The lower half of the table is a simulation of the effects on all of these of a period of growth-faltering. This starts sometime after the age of six months and by one year has transferred the growth path from the 50th down to the 5th percentile, which is then followed through to adulthood—a pattern typical of, for example, Indian farm-labor households.

If one looks simply at the difference in the daily cost of growth at the age of one year, this is a small saving, as Beaton (1989) says, of about 3 percent of the daily total. However, added to this instantaneous effect of growth-faltering is the cumulative reduction in total daily expenditure due to smaller size in addition to slower growth. Daily requirements at one year are 8 percent lower than for the child growing along the 50th percentile, 19 percent lower at 2 years and 31 percent lower at 10 years. Up to this age, the simulation assumes that the energy cost of physical activity is proportional to body weight. A 25-year-old Indian woman has a daily total expenditure rate 21 percent lower than an equally active woman of average (U.S.) body weight. If a realistic allowance were added for the effect of reduced body size in cutting the cost of productive work (here assumed to be 400 kilocalories per day irrespective of body size), reduction would be well over a quarter. Such a large weight reduction would, of course, be associated with some degree of stunting. However, such resistance to strain has to be adaptive in the limited sense that, without such stunting—and even making generous allowance for possible slightly higher earnings for taller people—the woman, if she were substantially taller, would be seriously wasted at her likely food intake; and severe wasting is a far greater threat to the lives of mother and fetus than moderate stunting.

Table 2—Energy savings and cumulative growth-faltering

Item	Age In Years						
	0	0.5	1	2	5	10	25
	Energy expenditure of girl in United States (NCHS 50th percentile)[a]						
Weight (kilograms)	3.2	7.2	9.5	11.9	17.7	32.5	57.0
Basal metabolic rate (kilocalories)	144	360	617	654	885	1,137	1,368
Activity (kilocalories)	113	224	317	401	584	705	847
Growth (kilocalories)	133	83	50	33	25	66	...
Total kilocalories/day	390	667	984	1,089	1,494	1,909	2,215
Lifetime kilocalories	...	32,000	81,000	446,000	1,760,000	4,860,000	16,360,000
	Energy expenditure of girl in India (NCHS 5th percentile after 6 months)[a]						
Weight (kilograms)	3.2	7.2	9.0	9.6	14.0	22.5	43.0
Basal metabolic rate (kilocalories)	144	360	585	528	700	788	1,032
Activity (kilocalories)	114	224	300	324	462	488	713
Growth (kilocalories)	133	83	22	33	17	33	...
Total kilocalories/day	391	667	908	885	1,179	1,309	1,745
Lifetime kilocalories	...	32,000	80,000	408,000	1,500,000	3,690,000	11,906,000
Kilocalories/day saved	...	...	77	204	315	600	470
			(8%)	(19%)	(21%)	(31%)	(21%)
Lifetime saving (kilocalories)	...	...	1,400	37,900	25,700	117,000	4,450,000

Source: Derived from pooled data from 95 studies published between 1914 and 1983; and P. R. Payne and M. Griffiths, private communications.
[a] NCHS is National Center for Health Statistics.

Even more striking than these quite substantial savings in daily energy needs are the cumulative savings of food energy over time. The bottom line of Table 2 shows that by the age of 25 these amount to 4,450,000 kilocalories, which is equivalent to seven years of food supply for an "Indian size" woman, or perhaps more strikingly, almost sufficient to provide for the food needs of another female individual up to the age of 10. This provides a second reason for attaching importance to lifetime energy-saving: moderately reduced child growth contributes to household resistance to strain. This could be usefully adaptive, even in the relatively short run. Household adaptations usually involve several adjustments. Any one of these, such as reduced growth rate by one member, while in itself contributing only a few percentage points to the reduction of total energy requirement, may be crucial to the household's accumulating enough total adjustment, or to its doing so at low or acceptable cost. In any case, there seems no reason to assume, as Beaton (1989) does, that the saving of energy consequent upon reducing the growth rate could be an effective adjustment *only* if the body had a mechanism for deploying it that was sensitive to a very small change in energy balance (such as the 2-3 percent equivalent to a single day's resulting saving of energy).

In assessing the claim that moderate stunting—undesirable as the process that causes it certainly is, and as the final state of shortness may perhaps be—constitutes an adaptive resistance to strain, both immediate and cumulative direct energy-saving effects on the individual must be taken together. In addition, the spin-off to others from the calories not consumed, summing up over all moments of time, provides the household with scope for adjustment to the same or other sources of stress.

Obviously, a number of biological mechanisms could be involved in bringing about these cumulative savings at the individual level. Probably the most important of these is the quite rapid decline, after the first year or so of life, in the growing child's capacity to make a full recovery of its original potential for growth in height. It is this progressive loss of the mechanism for complete catch-up that results in the accumulation of a permanent deficit in size and hence reduced energy needs. It seems unlikely that this pattern of relatively rapid loss of an initially effective mechanism of compensation would have survived the process of natural selection if it constituted a significant loss of biological fitness. The net advantage gained by individuals who were able throughout childhood and adolescence to maintain the path toward maximum achievable adult height (together with its strong correlates) must not in the past have usually exceeded the net advantage gained by individuals who experienced progressively inhibited child growth in response to energy stresses—despite the associated costs and dangers, including those of its strong correlates. Either Darwinian evolution resulting from natural selection is rejected or, in the absence of an alternative explanation, it has to be concluded that moderate reduction in child growth of height is usually an adaptive response, resisting strains caused by dietary energy stress. Whether such adaptation is seen to be *acceptable*, either in general or in particular instances, is another matter.

Similar considerations of the overall balance between gains and losses also apply to adult weight loss as an adjustment to energy stress.

Adjustments in both adults' body mass and children's rate of growth of height operate in two ways. First, as body tissues (energy stores) are burned up (or deposited more slowly), they release or save energy that is then available for the remaining body tissues, helping them to sustain function despite the reduction in food intake relative to requirements. All body tissues take some part in this response to energy stress but do so in proportions that reflect a strategy for survival, which is itself the result of natural selection in the past, the brain and nervous system being conserved with the highest priority. Second, because a smaller weight of body tissues remains (after adult body mass, or child growth of height, has been reduced), its total maintenance cost declines. Subsequently, the body can maintain energy balance with less food (or more work) than before.

The importance of both these direct responses to energy stress could be greatly altered if body size significantly affected any of three things: the makeup of the body, as between tissues with different initial resting metabolic rates; the specific metabolic rates under conditions of rest, per unit weight of any form of tissue; or the energy requirements for performing any sort of work or productive activity over and above the resting state. Discussions of these possible indirect consequences of body size adjustment are deferred to later sections of this chapter.

First, adjustment of body weight, or of growth of height in children, is examined as a two-part direct strategy: to slow down growth of (and, instantaneously, to mobilize) tissue to counter an immediate energy shortfall for other tissues; and to reduce body mass, and hence maintenance costs, to anticipate future energy shortfalls.

Differences in the relative involvement of fat and lean tissues in adjustments of body size are important in understanding the scope for such adaptation. Fat provides a relatively high density of energy storage that is deposited efficiently and contributes little to the cost of maintenance. In addition, the energy stored can be efficiently released with little risk of incurring any loss of physiological function (Dugdale and Payne 1987).[8] Unfortunately, groups at high risk of energy stress usually have little fat when it begins and indeed (Lee 1977) might be incommoded in their work if they had much more. Although the success of some agricultural populations in adapting to sharp seasonal stress does depend on the capacity to deposit and release a high ratio of fat to lean (Payne and Dugdale 1977), in other communities hunger causes its victims to lose weight with high lean content and thus to become "emaciated"—plainly a damaging response, although usually a reversible one.

The two time-series issues of the extent to which adult weight loss and child height growth retardation are adaptive responses to energy stress meet in the crosscutting question, Is low adult body size, of a person or group, compared with other persons or groups at the same period—and frequently due to some previous retardation of child

---

[8]This applies also to reduced rates of tissue deposition in children.

growth—to any extent an adaptive response to life in circumstances of chronic or repeated energy stress? The answer must depend to some extent on where one starts from. At-risk groups, such as the landless laborers examined by Shetty (1984), were already very thin (body mass index [BMI] values were below 16); so an even lower BMI, that is, further weight reduction, would involve considerable, though perhaps sometimes reversible, costs. But is a group of adults disadvantaged by having, on average, small achieved body size to the extent that, as is usual, this partly originated in some slowing down of growth in height during the early years of life? To decide whether small adult populations reflect previous child growth retardation that is itself adaptive or otherwise, the discussion must now revert to the issue of child growth relative to growth rates currently accepted for international comparisons: the NCHS standards, which are derived from measurements on U.S. population groups.

Growth of children in high socioeconomic categories in many other population groups for which data are available follows these NCHS growth curves rather closely (Keller and Fillmore 1983, 134). Although these authors carefully refrain from any such inference, this, together with the rapid secular increases in stature of both inter- and intra-population migrants, is often cited as evidence that (1) there are no significant genetic differences in the growth potential of different ethnic groups of humans. Those who are satisfied by such negative evidence often draw the further conclusion that (2) those large groups of adults, for example the populations of South India, who currently are on average smaller than Americans or Europeans, must be so not because they are constitutionally different but because they have adjusted their growth downward as a response to adverse environments. Although this is certain to be true, at least in part, it clearly does not exclude the possibility of underlying genetic differences.[9] Even less does it justify the frequent assertions that (3) such populations must not be described as "adapted," or that (4) even if adapted in the strictly Darwinian sense discussed earlier, they are not adapted acceptably because, being smaller than some normative size (such as the NCHS standard), they have not achieved their genetic potential. Still less is it proven that (5) even if genetic height potential had not been achieved, net disadvantage would result in the circumstances actually prevailing for such populations. Indeed, if the shortest people in many populations—comprising, probably, the poorest subpopulations—had grown to a greater adult height without improving their adult access to income and food, this would normally imply wasting.

These five propositions about genetic potential for attained height can be boiled down to two: (1) it can be assumed that a single mean value exists for maximum potential growth of stature and is applicable across all ethnic groups; and (2) important aspects of well-being, or of functional

---

[9]The genetic height potential of such groups may have been lower before adjustment than it is now; that is, adjustment may have eliminated carriers of genes that had earlier carried genetic potential for greater tallness.

efficiency of individuals, are always improved, the closer an individual approaches his or her genetically determined maximum stature, and hence growth performance.

The balance of evidence renders the first of these two propositions very dubious. To assimilate the growth performance of all populations to that of "high socioeconomic groups" excludes consideration of the most striking exceptions, namely, those relatively inbred tribal groups that still follow their traditional livelihoods. The achieved mean stature of such groups in Africa ranges between 144 centimeters for male Pygmies and 147 centimeters for the Bushmen of the southern Kalahari to 176.5 centimeters for the Tutsi (Barnicot 1964). This range is five times the standard deviation of adult male stature according to the NCHS standard. This may represent the maximum range of genetic differences among humans, since the current consensus is that indigenous African populations are the representatives of the oldest and hence most varied genetic pool, from which the ancestors of all other geographic/ethnic groups migrated comparatively recently. However, significant variations do exist elsewhere. A study of the growth of several tribes living in the highlands of New Guinea (Malcolm 1974) shows the mean stature of adult women as 12 centimeters shorter than that of European women and intertribal differences of 19 centimeters (3 standard deviations of the NCHS mean). While there are indeed very few people of that kind left alive, the populations of the Far East include a large majority of the world's people who are at risk of energy stress. Davies (1988) and Martorell (1985) quote studies on Japanese, Chinese, and Korean children whose growth approximates to the 25th percentile of the NCHS standard, even though they were living in relatively privileged environments.

Possibly, the motivation for denying the existence of genetic differences in potential height is concern for egalitarian rather than scientific principles. If so, it is foolishly misplaced. First, the existence (ideally to be continued) of morphological variance is a measure of the capacity of the species to respond to future new environmental stresses or opportunities. Second, in recent history, concern for genetic homogeneity seems more often to have led to authoritarianism than to increased regard for equality. Third, within-group variance (about the group mean for adult height) remains significant and is not thought to confer inequality. Fourth and above all, people are not giraffes. Tall is not, in general, beautiful. Tall or small may be adaptive or healthy, depending on environment.

In the Far East, particularly, people in almost wholly endogamous and largely very poor groups (notably agricultural labor castes in India) are often short in comparison with domestic high-income groups, and a fortiori with regard to the NCHS standards. Moreover, they are also thinner, being more than proportionately lower in body weight. Shetty (1984) reported that "poor Indian [adult male] labourers were able to work, and performed well in physiological tests, despite their thinness: they had BMI values (the ratio of weight in kilograms to the square of the height in meters) of 15-16 . . . and an estimated body fat content of 6 percent": respective U.S./European averages for men are around 23 and 20 percent, respectively (Waterlow 1989, 10). It is at least questionable whether such groups, even with total removal of childhood exposure to disease and dietary constraints, would achieve even the stature of well-to-do Indians, whose median height is at the 25th percentile of the NCHS level. Hereditary and endogamous castes of extremely poor laborers, surviving over many generations (and exemplifying the outcome of the process of natural selection), would presumably become not only smaller in body size but altered in other ways, such as body proportions and relative sizes of organs, so as to cope more effectively with low energy intakes and heavy work. If indeed such a group retained genetic potential for tallness, this could be expressed only via the emergence of recessive genes for tallness over several generations—after a change of environment that involved better prospects for food and work, and that thus moved the balance of advantage in favor of the emergence of these recessives, which had formerly been selected against (by mortality in the womb or in early life) in the harsher environments.

The alternative possibility is that the tallness genes have been so heavily selected against as to have been eliminated in these endogamous groups long accustomed to "hereditary" hardship. If so, such groups have a height potential lastingly adapted downward in order to survive, through reproduction of viable offspring, in their long-run environments. In that case, if the full achievement of genetic potential for growth is to be accepted as an objective of improved public health, it would seem necessary to admit the likelihood that not only each individual but every ethnic or other endogamous group mean has a different target to reach.

But what is the argument for the paramount objective of maximizing growth? In essence, it is the same as that which insists that no degree of individual adjustment of body size in response to environmental stress can be regarded as acceptable.

This report has already set out the argument that shifts in gene-environment interactions will always imply an altered balance of advantages and disadvantages. In face of prevailing or new circumstances, an adjustment (such as shifts to a below-maximum growth path) will not be durable in a population unless it sustains fitness, that is, unless as a result of adjustment the individual has improved or maintained, rather than diminished, its chances of contributing to the inheritance of future generations. It is contended here that the first need is to be able reliably to identify those people for whom even that condition has not been achieved. Achieving that priority, with reasonable assurance for all individuals in a society, in no way precludes subsequently "moving the goalposts" on the grounds that a second criterion should be addressed, namely of whether or not the condition of those who are still the worst-off is judged by the members of that society to be acceptable in regard to the ethical values currently prevailing. However, it is clear that this emphasis on the need to prioritize concerns also implies a shift, of the basis of policy, away from "goal-setting; problem solving; optimizing" toward the influence and management of "process," including not only the processes involved in adaptation but also those of the evolution of ethical standards.

The circumstances of many adults involve life with low or uncertain energy intakes; work requiring much body translation (and little heavy lifting); and hot, humid environments. Being considerably shorter and often somewhat thinner for height than richer or "Northern" populations, they may be more efficient in turning physical work into income and food as well as needing less, hence surviving better in their current environment. The selection process may partly be that children with genetically high energy needs have fewer survival prospects, but also partly that children consume somewhat low energy intakes relative to requirements and hence grow into smaller adults. Circumstances, such as persistent poverty, that eliminate many potentially viable and happy humans merely because they are large in body size and food needs are as a rule wholly deplorable. However, given these deplorable conditions, the result—low body size in adulthood—is not only a clear adaptation if it improves fitness but also is of itself not obviously deplorable. To establish that some specific degree of shortfall below a group's height potential (if demonstrable) was unacceptable, one would need to show that the subgroup of adults thus affected was disadvantaged in some way specifically related to their stature. An important dynamic example is that some ways out of poverty, for example via very heavy physical work such as lumberjacking, might be closed to populations that had adapted to poverty by means of very small stature and low BMIs.

Of course, if one were able to measure genetic potential in regard to some aspect of function almost universally valued, such as social competence or intelligence, then its full attainment would correctly be seen as a human right. In regard to height (and certainly to weight), however, this is not obvious, unless future research demonstrates that larger body size is a cause, not merely a statistical correlate, of some widely valued aspects of function.

Leaving aside this issue of the adaptiveness or undesirability of achieved adult size, what is the development cycle during which energy stress affects growth to adulthood, and which of the resultant strains are damaging? The impacts of supplementary feeding programs on the growth of children, even below six years of age, are much less than the theoretical increments implied by the amounts of supplement consumed (making corrections for losses, leakages, displacements, and so forth) (Beaton and Ghassemi 1982). Martorell, Klein, and Delgado (1980) showed that dietary supplements, contributing an average of 258 kilocalories and 18.2 grams per day while reducing the extent of height deficits of Guatemalan children at three years of age, still left them below the 5th percentile (–2 standard deviations below the mean) of the NCHS reference standard, although that standard is attained by the children of well-to-do Guatemalan families.[10]

Descriptions were presented earlier of how energy stress in very early life reduces growth, but relatively reversibly; how this potential for

---

[10]More recent work by Martorell, not yet published, suggests that by adolescence the supplemented children had still not caught up (J. R. Behrman, pers. comm.).

fully reversible responses is progressively reduced; and how the capacity of the mechanism of growth control to "reset" itself onto a lower track is a crucial response, not just to present but to expected future energy stress. Exactly at what age improving the diet or the health environment ceases to fully reverse the effects of early stress patterns on height growth is not known, but it is very early.

To some extent offsetting this limited capacity for catch-up between (say) 2 and 8 years or so in poor (energy-stressed) societies, and especially in poorer groups within them, the adolescent growth spurt is also effectively postponed. The result of this is that height gain between ages 12 and 18 is absolutely more than in better-off populations (Eveleth 1985, 32), though still much less than sufficient to bring mean height to the level of those populations (Ashworth and Millward 1986, 158). A capacity to delay growth until "the time is ripe" may itself be part of a selective adaptation to energy stress (Roberts 1985, 52). In the model shown earlier in Figure 1, this corresponds to the form of "tolerance of strain" that plant breeders call "latency." This renders some plants grown in semi-arid environments of variable rainfall, such as millet, better able to withstand moisture stress than plants adapted to less harsh environments, such as maize. Millets facing recurrent high risks of moisture stress—like some poor human populations similarly facing energy stress—have evolved the capacity to defer critical growth stages until conditions are more propitious.

While latency does counter some of the reduction of adult body size due to energy stress in childhood, some of that reduction remains. It is the overall outcome that forms part of a strategy of adaptation to adverse environments. More controversial is the question of whether the process is an acceptable adaptation.[11] Given that both short- and long-term responses are possible, what are the immediate costs of the process of becoming small, and what, if any, are the safe limits?

Much attention has been directed toward identifying associations between growth retardation in early life, aspects of performance such as resistance to infectious diseases, and cognitive development. The key question is the extent to which such associations provide evidence of causality. In reviewing the evidence, it is as well to keep firmly in mind the fact that growth retardation is itself a probable outcome of a wide variety of processes, including both disease and nutrition. In addition, many studies in the past have either explicitly or implicitly used current growth status as a measure of current or past nutritional status. Pelletier (1991) introduces his discussion of anthropometry and mortality thus: " . . . a distinction must be made between nutritional status and anthropometric

---

[11]It is not only energy intake, outgo, and metabolic rates that determine whether the amount of child growth, or of adult size reduction, remains in the "acceptable" range. Apart from vitamin B, iron, iodine, and some essential fatty acids, at least two micronutrients, zinc and vitamin A, play a catalytic role, as yet inadequately explored. And for a few populations with roots, tubers, or bananas as main staples, and with high energy requirements, "pure" shortage of protein may independently push size or growth below critical levels.

indicators of nutritional status, although the terms are sometimes used interchangeably . . . . Thus, the present review is concerned with anthropometry-mortality relationships in the first instance, and only through cautious inference does it discuss nutrition-mortality relationships." Osmani (1988, 56) summarizes the state of knowledge well. He contrasts the causative hypothesis that "moderate stunting does not impair any nutritionally determined capability" (here, Osmani is considering the hypothesis that there is *no* causality) with the associative hypothesis that "a moderately stunted child does not suffer from impairment of any nutritionally determined capabilities." He continues, "We feel inclined to treat the causative hypothesis sympathetically in view of our discussion of all the functions mentioned above. The associative statement however requires caution. We should not simply assume that a moderately stunted child is nutritionally sound, even if we accept the causative statement."

This casts a new light on the famous comment that "stunting can be seen as healthy only in the sense that scar tissue is healthy" (Martorell 1982). Citing this, Beaton (1985, 230) continues, "Small stature in a population is of concern because it is a marker of deprivation, not because smallness is bad in itself." Burning and child undernutrition are unhealthy; scar tissue is, and moderate stunting may be, the least unhealthy response available in many circumstances.

Moderate stunting without wasting is neither a cause nor a marker of current or *individual* deprivation. It is a marker, though not a cause, of previous *population* deprivation. All this seems to be agreed, despite the strong feelings and the rhetoric. Yet where smallness is in some part genetic, as for example is probably the case in most of South and East Asia, the deprivation thus marked, and the subsequent selection and competitive survival of smaller individuals, may have occurred millennia ago. If, on the other hand, there is unexpressed genetic potential for growth in a population, and if food shortage rather than disease is the current source of stress, what would be gained by only providing extra food to set children on the growth curves toward their maximum genetically attainable adult height and toward the NCHS median weight for that height? Obviously, without proportionally greater food supply as adults, they might well be faced by the need to repartition their work/time patterns away from tasks involving high levels of activity and toward tasks with lower energy cost but also lower productivity. Such children might therefore grow up to become poorer and hungrier and perhaps (at their taller heights) wasted. Without more physical activity in work or at leisure as adults, they could well grow up to be poor and fat. Circumstances of several "poor but overnourished" populations—for example, the upsurge of coronary heart disease in urban Sri Lanka, and of obesity among poor groups in many cases in the United States and even in Caribbean and West African urban areas—show that "poor and fat" is not just a hypothetical concern (Arteaga 1982; Ross and Minkowsky 1983; Stunkard and Singh 1972; see also Dugdale and Payne 1987). Both these sorts of adult populations—those generated by *only* feeding up children to attain full genetic growth potential, and hence poor and hungrier (perhaps wasted), and those that become fatter but remain poor—would be no more capable and no fitter than today's.

Risk of Death

There is general agreement that several indices of anthropometry are good predictors of subsequent mortality, certainly for those individuals whose growth is severely retarded. Sommers and Lowenstein (1975), Kielman and McCord (1978; see Lipton 1983a, 18), Chen, Chowdhury, and Huffman (1980), and Heywood (1982, 1986) have all demonstrated that a relationship exists between the anthropometric status of individuals and the likelihood of their dying subsequent to the measurement.

Pelletier (1991) has reviewed and reanalyzed the data from six of these studies, which cover a number of countries. This confirms that in all cases the relationship between the degree of deficit in body dimensions as compared with international reference standards and subsequent risk of mortality is highly significant and is nonlinear. With increasing size of growth deficit, mortality risk rises, at first rather slowly and then with increasing steepness as the deficits become greater. This is consistent for all anthropometric indicators, although as predictors of mortality, arm circumference and weight-for-age are much the most consistent and efficient, while height-for-age and weight-for-height are the poorest. While the general form of the relationship is consistent as between populations, the strength of the association is not. For a given deficit below the same (NCHS) mean in weight-for-age, South Asian children experience a much lower risk of death (2-4 times) than children in Africa or Papua New Guinea: an observation that casts serious doubt on the value of anthropometric indicators as measures for global comparison.

Pelletier (1991) disagrees with the interpretation of the form of the relationship given by Chen, Chowdhury, and Huffman (1980). This is that there exists a distinct "threshold" or breakpoint in the relationship that divides the range into two parts, with lower levels of growth deficit showing little if any association between size and the risk of death but higher deficits showing a strong positive correlation. Pelletier considers that the existence of a threshold is not supported by the cross-country analysis and that the data as a whole are better described by a continuous exponential function. However, with analyses of this kind, observations on individuals necessarily have to be aggregated into a limited number of groups in order to derive rates (of relative mortality). There are, as a result, in Pelletier's analysis only four data points covering the whole range that can be used to test the fit of any kind of model, exponential or otherwise. In addition, as Seckler and Young (1978) point out, when individual anthropometric data are aggregated, interindividual variation would conceal the location of any threshold point. The statistical power of Pelletier's analysis, even to distinguish between a "threshold" model (two intersecting straight lines) and an exponential curve, much less to reject the former, is, to say the least, questionable.

Drawing the "cautious inference" about the relationship between anthropometry and nutritional status, it seems plausible that the mechanism, which results in a nonlinear relationship between growth retardation and mortality risk, is itself due to a similar relationship between degree of immunocompetence and level of nutritional status, in which other deficiencies of vitamins or micronutrients such as zinc as well as protein-energy malnutrition (PEM) play a part. (This is discussed later in the section on resistance to infections.) The primary role of immuno-competence (or the lack of it), particularly in regard to severely growth-retarded children, is lent further plausibility by evidence of a strong positive effect of breast-feeding on their chances of survival. In two studies in Bangladesh, for example, the relative risk of mortality for the most severely, as compared with mildly, wasted children was between 5 and 10 times higher for weaned than for breast-fed individuals of the same age (Pelletier 1991). As in other studies (Butz, Habicht, and DaVanzo 1984) showing breast-feeding as a positive factor in reducing the mortality risk of poor sanitation or water supply, the benefit of breast-feeding appears to lie in its role as a source of maternal antibod-ies, reinforcing the immunological competence of the growth-re-tarded child, rather than in its nutritional properties.

Comparison of Heywood's (1986) results for Papua New Guinea with those of Chen, Chowdhury, and Huffman (1980) for Bangladesh suggests that the point on the scale of any anthropometric indicator above which children's risk of death begins to rise sharply may depend on the particular spectrum of infectious disease organisms to which they are exposed. With some reservations because of this, as well as of the possibility that the relationships are continuous (for example, exponen-tial) rather than discontinuous (threshold), the present study holds that there is a region of the scale of any anthropometric indicator below which individual children are likely to suffer much greater associated costs (in terms of mortality or permanent damage) than do those with smaller degrees of growth deficit. Furthermore, those costs are likely to rise much more steeply with any further decrements in growth. On available evidence, this point seems to be somewhere around the lower end of the range of individual variation found in well-to-do populations. It is common practice to use a level of two standard deviations (in the case of weight-for-age, about 20 percent of the mean) below the median value for well-to-do child populations to define the boundary between moderate and life-threatening malnutrition. However, it is also now clear that as measures of the limits of acceptable adjustment to nutri-tional stress, such conventional cut-off points should not be applied globally as a basis for policy. Being 20 percent below the mean for weight-for-age in the context of one particular pattern of infectious disease types and transmission processes might imply a tolerable, if not ideal, level of risk; in another context, the same growth status might involve very sharp rises in the risk of child death.

If the mean body sizes of adults are pushed to the left by adaptation, this may leave them "fit and well adapted" only at the cost of high child mortality (Crittenden and Baines 1985). This is almost certainly not, however, because of significantly higher risk of death among the children whose size would imply "mild" or "moderate" undernourishment. It is because, when the whole distribution of children aged 0-6 months, by height or by weight, is pushed to the left, a larger proportion of the children in the extreme left tail is severely undernourished. The rather small children will continue to survive into acceptably adapted adulthood.

Could reduced body size be counteradaptive by reducing the prospects of adult survival? The first point to consider is wasting, which alone is relevant to the adaptiveness, or otherwise, of adult body size reduction under energy stress (since height is already determined in adults). Extreme wasting is obviously harmful, but how much wasting is extreme? How much leanness is, instead, adaptive? Most of the direct evidence derives from developed countries. A prospective study of 1.9 million Norwegians (Waaler 1984) shows that the form of the relationship of BMI to general mortality experience is a U-shaped curve. There is a wide range of BMI values over which mortality risk is related only weakly, if at all, to BMI. That range is bounded at both extremes of BMI by a very steeply rising risk of mortality.

Values less than 18 or 19 for BMI in adult males seem to carry about 10 percent excess mortality risk—typically, a reduction in life expectancy of about three years (see also Cole, Gilson, and Olsen 1974). For women the curves are markedly steeper, which might suggest the need for a higher threshold value of between 19 and 20. The main causes of death associated with very low adult BMI values in Norway were tuberculosis, obstructive lung diseases, and lung and stomach cancer (Waaler 1984, 31).

However, it cannot be inferred that, even in Norway, BMI below 18-20 "causes" higher mortality. First, both tuberculosis and very low adult BMI are known to be caused in part by child and adult poverty and its consequences. Second, and more important, this study made no distinction between smokers and nonsmokers. Smoking causes both greatly reduced life expectancy and reduced BMI in smokers and in their children—once again explaining part of Waaler's finding, even if low BMI does not cause higher mortality. Third, there is a likelihood that some of the low BMI readings are caused by as yet undiagnosed cases of wasting disease, even though invalids, persons in hospitals, and those already under control or treatment for tuberculosis were excluded (Waaler 1984, 8-9).

An especially worrying possibility, in view of the rapid spread of cigarette smoking among poor people in such developing countries as China (where it is expected to cause 2 million deaths yearly by the early 2000s [Commission on Health Research 1990, 14]), is that BMI below 18-20 may somehow increase the risk from smoking. There is some evidence for this harmful synergism (P. James, pers. comm.). Hundreds of millions of adults in poor countries will continue to have BMIs well below these 18-20 borderlines. The spread of cigarette smoking there could in future turn body-size reduction from an adaptive response to energy stress into a hidden further cause of death.

Actuarial data also show that mortality in middle-aged U.S. males from various occupations is higher for those with BMIs below 19 (Keys 1980). For British men aged 55-65 (Cole, Gilson, and Olsen 1974), mortality rates were three times higher for the group with BMIs below 19.7 than for those between 19.7 and 22.4. (They were twice as high as for those above 22.4.) However, these U.K. and U.S. data, unlike the Norwegian, do not exclude low-BMI hospital populations, many of whom have low BMI because they are seriously ill. Also, the U.K. and U.S. (like the Norwegian) data are affected by inclusion of nonhospitalized cases in which early stages of disease are caused by low BMI (or caused simultaneously with it) or by adverse childhood health environments, rather than by the concurrent effects of low BMI itself. Furthermore, the greater prevalence of smoking, low BMI, and lung cancer and obstructive lung diseases among the poor—nutrition apart—applies to these data as well as to the Norwegian data.

Moreover, the causes of excess mortality in low-BMI persons in Norway are not main causes of adult deaths in India (except for tuberculosis, which itself causes low BMI). It is not known whether BMIs of 16-19 (apparently consistent with health among Indian agricultural laborers [Shetty 1984]) in fact raise mortality risk in poor tropical populations; these have much lower mean BMIs than in Norway, and higher overall mortality, but of course quite different sets of health hazards. It is hoped that future research will analyze relationships of BMI to age-specific mortality for populations and subgroups in poorer countries. Populations that have lower mean adult BMIs probably will also have lower levels of BMI (for each sex) below which age-specific death rates start to rise sharply. For small children, that is suggested by the evidence cited earlier in this section. For adults, there are straws in the wind—no more—to support such a hunch. One such straw, to the extent that illness rates predict mortality rates, is a study of 199 men in Bangladesh; their risk of illness rose sharply with low BMI, but only when BMI fell below 17 (Pryer 1990).

The steeply rising risk of death associated with very high values of BMI may well be relevant to the adaptive success, or acceptability, of low BMIs even in very poor populations if these are likely to become richer and if a major concern is to avoid the spread of "diseases of affluence" as they do so. Like low BMI, high BMI is also a "marker" of earlier events that increase risks to life and health; hence the current concern about overnutrition in richer populations. The problems of being overweight, such as hypertension, diabetes, and heart disease, are well reviewed elsewhere. There is, in addition, a substantial body of evidence from animal studies suggesting that rapid growth in early life (and maximum body size) is associated with early onset of degenerative diseases (and early death). A review by Pariza (1987) concentrates particularly on cancer risk. Pointing out that calorie restriction is one of the most effective ways to decrease cancer risk in animals, Pariza notes the growing emergence of epidemiological evidence for similar relationships in man, especially in combination with sustained high levels of energy expenditure.

All this suggests major risks, especially to steadily aging populations, of insisting now upon apparently "safe" high thresholds for energy intakes in early life, predefining the growth of children into pathways that imply possibly ill-advised levels of energy requirements later on. This could be an important consideration in defining nutrition policies, especially in the developing areas of Asia and Latin America (though not, as yet, in most of Africa), which have a clear prospect of an aging population.

Those who see the value of requirements as primarily prescriptive—and who therefore do not accept adaptations that reduce body size and hence cut down requirements—need to bear in mind that obesity arises very rapidly in populations that, even if not aging rapidly, acquire even quite modest levels of improved food supply and leisure. Obesity as a cause of increased death risk associated with poverty, not affluence, in the United States—especially among ethnic groups adapted until recently to survive heavy farmwork on low energy intakes—is a warning sign for poor populations in "successful" developing countries. So is the serious rise since 1945 in obesity-related degenerative diseases in Sri Lanka. Early formation of more (or, less riskily, of larger) fat cells among children in societies not providing extra income-earning activity in later life could be a tragic and ironic upshot of inaccurately identifying and "treating" populations of the alleged marginally undernourished.

Clearly, BMI in adults can lead to higher death risk by being too low or too high; for BMI (as for weight), an approach to genetic potential is itself unacceptable. What of height? Several studies, notably that already mentioned of Norwegian adults by Waaler (1984), show an independent relationship between final height and general mortality experience. The relationship is positive, that is, life expectancy increases with tallness throughout the range of stature (with some evidence of a reversal only for the extremely tall). However, shortness could well be associated with BMI, not as a direct cause, but due to the associations with poverty and smoking by parents and children, leading to subsequent smallness and high risk of lung disease when the children grow up. Just as smallness in children may be best thought of as a retrospective marker for the effects of environmental stresses in very early life, so it seems that some of those early events continue throughout life to exert a lasting effect both on the course of growth in stature and on susceptibility to the effects of disease and other stresses.

If this is correct, secular upward trends in adult height would be expected in the populations of developing countries, accompanied by reduced mortality from general causes. This would mirror the changes seen in developed countries over the past few generations. At the moment, it cannot be said how differences in genetic potential for height, as between South Asians and Norwegians, for example, will influence the speed or magnitude of such changes.

Nor is it certain that, say, a 20-year program to help South Asian children to grow closer to their genetic potential for adult height—in the absence of better economic prospects for those adults—would raise adult life expectancy. Suppose that an onslaught on mild-to-moderate child stunting led to a substantial increase in adult height, yet adults then had the same degree of command over food. Adult weight-for-height would then fall well below levels that would have prevailed in the absence of the height increase. This, in turn, would probably lead to a general upward impact on adult mortality risk. At very low incomes, moderate stunting may be the only feasible alternative to wasting, which is usually more dangerous. Thus, concern that some plausible food policies might make, say, India's poorest groups little or no better off on average—and at the extremes (in the right tail of their body-size distributions) dangerously fat, tall, or large, or (in the left tail for BMI) at greater risk from adult wasting than they used to be from moderate stunting—is not as absurd as might at first appear.

However, even if rather small average height of adults in many populations is a successful adaptation, mainly because it reduces risks of adult death in energy stress, it is often "bought" with a severely malnourished left tail of the height-for-age distribution of preschoolers. Children in this tail are at significantly increased risk of death. Special care for these maladaptive children matters more than feeding-up of the less severely malnourished.

Resistance to Infections

Two reviews (Martorell 1985; Tomkins and Watson 1989) reach similar conclusions about the effects of growth impairment on children's infections. First, regarding the incidence (that is, the frequency with which children with different levels of growth performance suffer illness) of measles, diarrhea, and pneumonia, there seems to be no relationship between incidence rates and anthropometry over a major part of the range of anthropometric measurements (see also Martorell and Ho 1984) except for the possibility that growth deficits caused in the first place by measles may be subsequently followed by increased susceptibility to diarrhea (Tomkins 1981). There is, however, some suspicion of increased rates of incidence of diarrhea in severely growth-affected children.

Regarding severity of illness, the evidence seems to point to no, or only slight, differences between normal and mildly growth-retarded individuals, but very markedly worse effects on the severely undergrown, particularly for the important childhood diseases such as measles and diarrhea. The one important exception to this pattern seems to be that of duration of the infection for diarrhea: even moderate growth reduction is associated with an extension of the duration of symptoms. However, this is directly related to earlier impairment of immunocompetence, not mediated by current nutritional status (Koster et al. 1987), and thus to earlier severe undernutrition. Moderate stunting (Bhaskaram et al. 1980) appears to have little affect on overall immunocompetence or its components, whereas severe stunting does (Osmani 1988, 46). The evidence and diagrams in Chandra (1981, 1991) also indicate impaired immunocompetence from upper-moderate and severe stunting, but to a much lesser extent at "marginal" levels. Martorell (1985, 22) summarizes in this way: "In a nutshell, nutrition seems to have little to do with *who* gets sick. On the other hand, more studies indicate an association between nutritional status (anthropometry) and the severity of infections." But in most of these studies it is wasting, seldom stunting and hardly ever moderate stunting, that is thus associated (Osmani 1988, 45).

It looks as if moderate stunting does not, as a rule, make infections more frequent, prolonged, or serious. Indeed, "depression of the immune system is observed regularly in clinical malnutrition symptoms caused by multiple nutrition deficiencies," especially of zinc, iron, and vitamin A (Buzina et al. 1989, 174). However, a serious problem, recognized by these reviews, is that most of the studies show positive relationships between illness and undernutrition (or, at any rate, anthropometric shortfalls) but do not clarify the causal sequence. Thus Belkenchir et al. (1985, esp. p. 91) show a strong relationship between diarrheal frequency (though not incidence) and simultaneous weight-for-age, which might be cause or effect of illness. However, they find no link between birth weight and subsequent probability of suffering diarrhea on any randomly selected day.

Much less is known about the impact of anthropometry on adult risks of illness and infection. A study by Pryer (1990) of 199 fathers of malnourished children aged under five years in Bangladesh showed that, whereas 44 percent of those with BMIs of less than 16 (and 33 percent with BMIs between 16 and 17) had lost labor days in the preceding month, a much lower proportion (10-12 percent) of those with values between 17 and 20 lost employment time. Once again, severe anthropometric impairment is indicted as unacceptable because it carries a high risk of infectious illness, whereas lesser impairment does not (compare Chen, Chowdhury, and Huffman 1980 on child death risk, also for Bangladesh).

Cognition

Concerning mental development, there is almost certainly a level of deprivation in very early life, associated with severe wasting, at which some irreversible damage is done to brain functions (Brozek 1979). For milder or later episodes, problems of measurement, and of correcting for confounding factors, are very severe. Some of the most extensive studies involving a food intervention have been made in Guatemala (Barrett, Radke-Yarrow, and Klein 1982). Food supplements were made available to women during pregnancy and lactation, and subsequently to their offspring. This was done on a voluntary basis, subjects being given food on request at health centers. The amounts of food taken varied considerably, but it is said that there were no differences between the high and low uptake groups in terms of household socioeconomic status. The outcomes were measured in terms of physical growth, morbidity, and a wide range of tests of cognitive development and of social interactive behavior of the children and, on later follow-up, subsequent school performance. The results show that on average the growth and behavioral performance, measured in terms of spontaneous exploratory levels, competitiveness, persistence, and so forth, of the children were poorer for the boys but not the girls in the group whose uptake of supplementary food was smaller. At the age of six to eight years, these children continued to show greater passivity, lower levels of play activity, and more dependence on adults.

Even if such differences later vanish and do not affect performance in cognitive tests, as appears to be the case (Valenzuela 1988) except in severe earlier undernutrition, while they last they are probably unpleasant for the children. This shows that being in the low-uptake group, which was not lower in income, is not acceptable. However, even if these features of the low-uptake children were indeed the results of damage due to undernutrition rather than to continued subsequent exposure to poor environments, it is difficult to see what are the practical implications of a trial that shows that low voluntary acceptance of food supplements is associated with subsequent poor performance. Moreover, damage was not reflected in school performances after three years at school (see sources cited by Lipton 1983a, 17); in mildly and moderately stunted primary school children, intellectual growth appears to "catch up" with their taller colleagues.[12]

Moderate stress leading to moderate degrees of stunting, given normal stimulation, may delay learning or socialization at school, but has not been at all persuasively shown to cause any long-term decline or shortfall in mental performance on its own. "Small bodies maintain a low but statistically significant correlation with comparatively low intelligence test scores and low school achievement" (Buzina et al. 1989, 175) for reasons similar to those explaining why "taller children are more likely to enroll in school earlier" (Pollitt 1990, 90). Such correlations reflect (1) the relationship over the whole range, including extreme smallness that does confer cognitive disadvantage, and (2) the effects of a process of becoming small, not necessarily the drawbacks of moderately small attained size, which in itself can be largely or wholly overcome by "positive deviance" in child care (Zeitlin, Mansour, and Bajrai 1987).

Except for severe undernutrition, "big is smart" only to the extent that high income tends to facilitate education, stimulation, and food intake to attain bigness, and perhaps selection of genes for it (Osmani 1988, 53-55). For 2,300 randomly selected grades 1-4 pupils in the Philippines, in a regression model allowing for "pupil, school, teacher, and family variables . . . energy intake was found to be a significant predictor of school attendance, but [not] of overall test score and scores in local standardized tests in mathematics and reading" (Florencio 1989). Slightly subnormal energy intake relative to requirements, and its possible results among children in terms of mild-to-moderate stunting without wasting, are—in populations where their incidence is high—"markers," in Beaton's (1989) words, that many such children are in households too deprived to care for them properly. As this deprivation is remedied, children's food intakes and requirements will increase, along with their school performance and their physical growth rates. But these rates on their own are effects, not causes, of poverty.

Size and Work Capacity

Adaptation to energy stress via reduced child growth, and hence lower adult body size, is clearly not acceptable if smallness in adulthood imposes a significantly less satisfactory choice of work or a significantly higher cost (for example, risk of serious occupational illness) for making an otherwise satisfactory choice. Unfortunately, the literature is very confusing, partly because many different indicators of adult body size are used: height, weight-for-height, BMI (w/h^2), lean body mass, and

---

[12]In fact, these differences in behavior were seen for the most part in boys rather than girls.

others. In what follows, "large" and "small" are rather loosely used to cover all these indicators, but distinctions are attempted where necessary. The bioengineering aspects of how body size affects adult working capacity seem to be fairly clear.

There is considerable evidence of a significantly positive relationship between adult body size and maximum physical work capacity. As a proxy for maximum physical work capacity, physiologists use an indicator of the maximum aerobic capacity or maximum rate of oxygen uptake, VO_2max. VO_2max is a measure of the maximum rate of oxidation of energy-yielding substrate that an individual can attain in the short term.

It is useful to think of total-body VO_2max as the product of body weight and aerobic capacity per unit of body weight (that is, VO_2max per kilogram). The most significant determinants of VO_2max per kilogram are the health of the circulatory system and the level of habitual physical activity. However, body weight (kilograms) accounts for over 80 percent of the differences in total-body VO_2max among subjects suffering from varying degrees of protein-energy malnutrition (Spurr and Reina 1989). Since stunted adults are likely to have less body mass than adults of normal height, they are also likely to have lower VO_2max on that account.

In view of the major role of weight in determining VO_2max, it is hardly surprising that numerous studies have found high correlations, not only between body size and VO_2max, but also between each of these and measures of productivity. Spurr (1984) found that larger and taller Colombian workers were able to cut and load more sugarcane tonnage in a given time than were other workers. Brooks, Latham, and Crompton (1979) found that men with higher weight-for-height took less time to complete tasks such as wheelbarrow work, ditch digging, and earth excavation. Immink et al. (1984) found that the fat-free mass of Guatemalan wage laborers correlated linearly with the amount of coffee beans picked per day, the amount of sugarcane cut and loaded, and the speed of weeding a given surface area. Thus Spurr (1984) concluded that, in occupations involving heavy physical work, stunted workers will have lower productivity (output per person per hour).

However, except in particular circumstances of employment or of time allocation, differences among persons in physical output per hour (given the task, technique, and end-product) need not imply differences in value added, or in earnings, per person. Duration of work of given intensity, type of task, method of working—all can be adapted to body size. Therefore, the physical capacity to produce does not depend simply on VO_2max, but also, given VO_2max, upon endurance, that is, the fraction of VO_2max that can be sustained over time; the requirements of a particular task for a specific rate of work, given a particular body size; and ergonomic factors affecting task efficiency. Hence smaller people can sometimes adapt by choosing different working durations or intensities, tasks, or ergonomic patterns. Only if all this leaves small people in receipt of less income than large people, after allowing for the lower food requirements of smaller bodies, or if small people are compelled to do more work or less-preferred kinds of work for a comparable income, could one consider the adaptation through reduced height as possibly unacceptable through its impact on the work process. Even then, because poorer people tend also to be smaller people, one would need to inquire whether it was poverty (and therefore lack of skills and education), or smallness as such, that led to the concentration of small people in less satisfactory lines of work.

Where poor people must specialize in very heavy work, such as cane-cutting, at fixed time-rates of pay, they are clearly at a disadvantage if they are small; that is, employers are likely to select against them or to pay them less per hour or both.[13] This is partly offset by the lower amount of food that small people need to buy (although poor people in less-developed countries typically spend over 70 percent of income on food). However, given the empirical nature of the relationship of shortness to muscle mass, it cannot be assumed that short people are any worse at even heavy physical work than others (Osmani 1988). Why? Lower productivity in a given task may be offset by greater endurance, longer and slower work, or selection of less heavy physical tasks, in which short or lean adults have advantages.

Although small people, as measured by weight, height (if it proxies lean body mass), BMI, or weight-for-height, have lower VO_2max than "large" but non-obese people, body size is not associated with reduced VO_2max per unit of lean body mass. This, given the level of "training effect," is constant regardless of body size (Viteri 1971; compare Spurr and Reina 1989, 15, 18). Ferro-Luzzi (1985), using data from 36 countries, found that VO_2max per kilogram did not decrease as anthropometric indicators varied between normal levels and those that are usually taken to indicate mild or moderate undernourishment.

Indeed, sometimes marginally malnourished boys have higher VO_2max per kilogram than others (Barac-Nieto, Spurr, and Reina 1984), indicating one or more of the following: training effect in the narrow sense, that is, higher VO_2max per kilogram of muscle mass, given the level of muscular efficiency; higher muscle-mass/body-weight ratios; and higher muscular efficiency. This last possibility is exemplified by differences in average energy expenditure between normal and undernourished Colombian boys in a series of tasks, as measured by Spurr (1984); "the advantage of low body weight amounts to about 0.08 kcal per minute for each kg." These biological possibilities at work arise before even considering behavioral options, such as ergonomically greater task efficiency—units of task done per unit of work (energy expenditure)—by poorer persons with less total muscle mass, to whom energy-saving is more important. The biological options above all probably result from bodily changes due to past work, transport, and recreation patterns, all associated with poverty or smallness.

Indeed, where heavy, lifting-type physical work is not involved, so VO_2max matters less, smallness can confer energy advantages (less body weight to move to, from, or at work). If smaller (or poorer) workers nevertheless have lower output per hour than others, even at moderate

---

[13]This and the next sentence can easily be reinterpreted for circumstances of self-employment; there is no major change in the conclusion.

or light work, that is likely to be associated with specific deficiencies, especially of iron, and not with mild to moderate protein-energy malnutrition, past or present. In female Indian plantation workers, tea plucked per month was significantly related to hemoglobin (grams per deciliter of blood) but not to anthropometric measurements. Iron supplements alone improved both hemoglobin levels and productivity (Chaliha Kalita and Seshadri 1989, 314).

Another useful way to analyze the adaptations of work to body size (and hence, in part, to nutritional stress) is to point out that sustainable working output depends on (1) VO_2max; (2) the proportion of VO_2max at which a person can work for a given prolonged period, say four or eight hours; (3) the efficiency of conversion during this period to kilocalories of work done per 100 kilocalories of energy expenditure; and (4) ergonomic efficiency in converting work into economic product. This behavioral adjustment is discussed in Chapter 6, but even through biological variation alone—since (2) typically ranges from 20 percent to 40 percent and (3) from 15 percent to 25 percent—there is plenty of scope for adults with low VO_2max (for example, small adults) to produce as much physical work output as large adults, even at heavy work. This could be done by one of the following methods.

First, small workers could increase the physical intensity of work above that for large workers. Studies have shown that even an 8-hour day of heavy work seldom requires more than 35-40 percent of VO_2max of the individual (Michael, Hutton, and Horvath 1961; Åstrand 1967). By performing, say, at 40 percent of VO_2max where a large adult performs at 35 percent, a small adult could perform heavy work at the same productivity level. The cost of performing at this higher level of physical intensity, as in fact the smaller worker in general does, is that his or her heart rate is higher while working than the heart rate of a comparably "trained" large worker (Satyanarayana, Nadamuni Naidu, and Narasinga Rao 1979; see also Crabbe 1783). Hence small workers, given the same muscular efficiency, would have a higher energy cost per kilogram of performing heavy work, partly offsetting the energy savings from their lower body weights.

Second, as suggested above, this can be offset by training effect on the cardiovascular system. If small workers continue to perform heavy work at a higher physical intensity relative to large workers, this effect gradually raises not only the efficiency of their muscles other than the heart, but also—even assuming constant efficiency of muscles apart from the heart itself—the physical effect that workers can exert at a given heart rate (Satyanarayana, Nadamuni Naidu, and Narasinga Rao 1979; Barac-Nieto, Spurr, and Reina 1984). Thereby energy costs to small workers are reduced. This increase in the pumping capacity of the heart muscle—its efficiency in processing oxygen, that is, true training effect—is distinct from the effect of any change in body composition (for example, rising muscle-fat ratio). Rather it must reflect a higher oxidative capacity of muscle cells among those workers who have gone through the training effect. Nevertheless, large children perform several sets of tasks with less effort than small children (Barac-Nieto, Spurr, and Reina 1984).

In short, small adults must work at a higher physical intensity or rely to a greater extent on training effect, or both, in order to perform work involving heavy lifting, pushing, or pulling of external objects; but work involving relatively little of that, and a lot of movement of one's own body, can be done more efficiently by small adults than by large adults. A small boy expends less energy in moving his body than a large boy (Spurr et al. 1983). Also, small adults typically have much more lean per unit of fat than heavy adults of similar height, but not very different skeleton weight. This reduces small adults' energy cost per unit of muscle mass of moving their own bodies (Barac-Nieto, Spurr, and Reina 1984) and also reduces discomfort and distress associated with fatness when people work in humid heat (Lee 1977).

The upshot is that small (lean, short) persons are at an advantage in work requiring mainly body translation, where their low fat-lean ratio reduces "wasted effort," while their lower discomfort levels—and possibly higher VO_2max per kilogram—increase endurance. However, small persons are at a disadvantage in work requiring mainly heavy lifting, and so forth, where their low total muscle mass and low total VO_2max reduce performance.

So much for work-linked consequences of body-size adaptation within a given generation. Many generations of hard work, under energy stress, may also result in genetic selection, not only for size, but also for body build. Wade, Marbut, and Round (1990) have shown that leanness in men is associated with a high ratio of slow-twitch to fast-twitch muscle fibers—wholly a genetic characteristic. Since slow fibers are comparatively well endowed with mitochondria, the implication is that, other things being equal, low-BMI individuals will tend to have higher values of VO_2max per kilogram of lean tissue than will high-BMI individuals. A related issue is that small, but otherwise healthy, adults appear to perform steady, continuous tasks at "higher absolute mechanical efficiency," that is, they convert a higher proportion of the work done by muscle contraction into useful work done on the environment (lifting, pulling, levering, and so forth). At lower rates of work, this implies a lower total oxygen consumption for doing the same amount of work as a larger person. However, their "delta mechanical efficiency," that is, the additional energy cost of each increment of work load, is not superior, so that for increasingly heavy tasks the larger muscle mass of bigger people puts them at an advantage (Satyanarayana and Someshwar Rao 1989).

Whether the biological consequences for work performance of mild to moderate stunting (and even perhaps of mild wasting) are acceptable adaptations to energy stress, in relation to their impact (after full adjustment) upon adult size and hence working capacity, depends on non-biological considerations. Specifically, such consequences are unacceptable if, and only if, entire communities of low mean height or weight, or small individuals within communities, specialize in forms of work where smallness confers a net disadvantage and cannot change that specialization without significant loss to themselves, to others, or to the process of economic development and poverty reduction. Is this the case?

For individuals, Satyanarayana et al. (1977) and Satyanarayana, Nadamuni Naidu, and Narasinga Rao (1979) collate evidence that lower adolescent and adult weight is associated with lower wage rates, lower total work output in agricultural tasks, and presumably specialization in lower-paid tasks, but that lower height alone is not so correlated. The weight correlation probably does reflect employers' preference for people with higher (lean) body mass as well as the correlation of poverty to both mild-to-moderate undernutrition and low wage rates. Absence of a height correlation, however, suggests that—notwithstanding childhood stunting—subsequent improved nutrition, plus training effect, can build muscle and restore normal earning capacity.[14] The evidence that early undernutrition, even if it leads only to mild or moderate reduction in adult height, causes maladaptive changes in work capacity—and that adults cannot respond to such changes in ways that avoid overt damage—seems quite unpersuasive.

Overt damage, yes. But the vigorous attempt made here to give logical coherence to the confused and difficult subject of workers' adaptation to energy stress is not entirely satisfactory. Both the economics and the natural science, at the levels both of theory and of evidence, indeed suggest that the alleged physical and income drawbacks of moderate smallness-at-work are themselves very small. But some of the adaptations reviewed here tend to be very unpleasant. Harder, longer, work; more endurance; higher heart rates; and reliance on training effect, which is lost with a couple of weeks of bed rest, so that quite minor illness can greatly, even if only briefly, reduce subsequent working capacity: even if survival and income are not much affected, what a life! Crabbe's (1783) description of farmworkers in eighteenth-century rural England serves as a useful warning against undue "adaptation optimism" about undernutrition, and not only in regard to work performance. The most relevant lines—poetic, but (for example, in their closing observation of anorexia) far from unscientific—include

> Or will you deem them amply paid in health,
> Labour's fair child, that languishes with wealth?
> Go then! and see them rising with the sun,
> Through a long course of daily toil to run;
> See them beneath the dog-star's raging heat,
> When the knees tremble and the temples beat . . .
> See them alternate suns and showers engage,
> And hoard up aches and agues for their age . . .
> Then own that labour may as fatal be
> To these thy slaves, as thine excess to thee . . .
> There you may see the youth of slender frame
> Contend with weakness, weariness and shame;
> Yet, urged along, and proudly loth to yield,
> He strives to join his fellows of the field:
> Till long-contending nature droops at last,
> Declining health rejects the poor repast . . . .

---

[14]There is a limit to the extent of smallness that can be "compensated for" by the greater training effect in reducing heart rate at a given work level derived by small persons from regularly achieving a given level or VO_2. Extremely small adults ("severely undernourished") show a significantly higher heart rate at 40 percent of their own VO_2max than do other groups. Controls, mildly undernourished, and moderately undernourished groups show no significant differences (Spurr 1984, 231, diagram 10c).

Changes in Body Composition

Adjustment of body-fat stores is the most obvious component of the response to changes in energy intake, either in an upward or downward direction. It is not always appreciated that such changes are inevitably linked to some extent with changes of lean tissue as well. Studies of partial or total starvation show that, as fat stores are mobilized, there is always some loss of lean body mass (Payne and Dugdale 1977). However, the fact that more fat than lean is lost—given that fat has lower BMR per kilogram than lean—represents a maladaptive effect when taken in isolation: total-body BMR per kilogram rises somewhat, reducing the amount of energy saved by the weight reduction. Undernourished children probably show reduced skeletal muscle tissue (as well as reduced fat) relative to high BMR per kilogram organ tissues, accounting for their "perversely" raised sleeping metabolic rate per kilogram as compared with well-nourished controls (Vasquez-Velasquez, Prentice, and Coward 1989, 421).

The proportion of energy mobilized from fat, as compared with lean, varies quite widely from one individual to another. If very little fat has been stored, obviously little can be mobilized (this is yet another reason why women, with their higher fat-lean ratios, usually tolerate energy stress better than men). Damage is normally reduced if fat can be mobilized, for three main reasons: it is more dispensable than lean, the cost of mobilizing it is less, and the energy released per kilogram metabolized is much greater than from lean tissue.[15] This easily outweighs the maladaptive effect, just discussed, that mobilization of fat (rather than lean) raises RMR per kilogram.

When a transient fall in body weight is reversed and energy stores are replenished, the various body tissues increase in weight in nearly the same proportions as they had previously decreased. Therefore the continual swings between positive and negative energy balance, which are a normal part of existence, do not lead to cumulative changes in body composition. Payne and Dugdale (1977) suggest that the range of interindividual variation is from 97 percent of energy stored as fat and 3 percent as lean, to 70 percent as fat and 30 percent as lean, with a median value of 85 percent and 15 percent. They also suggest that a propensity to use and replace fat as an energy store, rather than relying on depletion of lean body mass, is a useful adaptation of population groups to situations in which food supply and energy expenditure fluctuate throughout the agricultural production season. A population

---

[15]"In man, short-term fluctuations of energy balance probably occur all the time, in [day-night] rhythm, and his body appears to be well equipped to mobilise stored energy. Body fat [is] a specialised organ, capable of correcting energy imbalance in the short term . . . as one of the early . . . physiological responses of the body. Serial [weight] data therefore should be an excellent operational indicator . . . of adaptation mechanisms at work, in the context of seasonality" (Ferro-Luzzi, Pastore, and Sette 1988, 37).

that is adapted to subsistence agriculture would be likely to comprise a high proportion of "fat storers," although their year-round average weights would be low in relation to height.

However, if such people—that is, lean people with a high propensity to store extra weight as fat—began to make use of a less energy-using range of production possibilities, perhaps with mechanical aids or following a move to an urban environment, body weights would increase, with the addition of a high proportion of fat. This is consistent with the known, large genetic component to obesity and with the phenomenon of rapidly increasing prevalence of obesity during urbanization. Little is known about changes in the proportions of nonfat tissues in response to changes in intake, although such changes do occur. Some organs, such as the liver, function as short-term "buffer" stores, smoothing out the intermittent flow of nutrients. The effects of relative changes of weight of some of the more metabolically active tissues such as liver, gut, heart, and kidney on the whole-body metabolic rate could be substantial and difficult to distinguish from effects due to alteration of metabolic efficiency.

There is little in the literature on body composition in field conditions that can also be linked to socioeconomic factors. In Papua New Guinea, highland men had greater body weights and fat-free masses than most coastal men, but stature, body density, skinfold thicknesses and fat mass were similar in the two groups (Norgan, Ferro-Luzzi, and Durnin 1982). Among the Masai in East Africa, significantly greater variances for the skinfold measurements in nontribals compared with tribals were found, suggesting that a redistribution of body fat accompanied the transition from tribal to nontribal states (Day, Bailey, and Robinson 1979).

Changes in Specific Metabolic Rates of Tissues: Metabolic Adaptation

A reduction in BMR is an invariable feature of prolonged energy deficiency. Much of it is the result of a decrease in active tissue mass. Under conditions of prolonged semistarvation, the RMR per kilogram is also substantially reduced, by as much as 20 percent (Keys et al. 1950). There is general agreement that the costs of adjustment to this extent are severe and unlikely to be acceptable in general (as distinct, of course, from the particular case of bearing those costs and surviving starvation longer, as distinct from refusing to pay them and dying sooner). However, adjustments of a smaller extent than these in the metabolic activity per unit weight of lean tissues are certain to occur as a component of "normal" intraindividual variability (Shetty et al. 1987, 33).

There has been continuous speculation and dispute about the magnitude of this "smaller extent" during the past few years. Once again, the dispute is intensified by those who take the view that no adjustment that incurs a demonstrable cost of any kind or degree can be described as adaptive. The "normal" range of variation, from day to day, of BMR per kilogram within an individual probably lies somewhere between 2 and 4 percent (see the comprehensive review by Millman and Chen 1991). However, there is little experimental evidence about the costs incurred by individuals who make adjustments in the range intermediate between this and the 20 percent reductions displayed by the subjects of semistar-vation experiments (Keys et al. 1950); hence there is no basis for judgments about their acceptability or otherwise. There is certainly no theoretical reason for assuming that changes greater than 2-4 percent in the specific metabolic rates of tissues cannot take place without cata-strophic or permanent loss of integrity. This would not contravene any of the laws of thermodynamics, nor would it require any revision of our present view of how energy is transformed in biological systems. There is nothing in the way metabolism is regulated in the whole body that dictates a constant efficiency of conversion.

In fact, there appears to be plenty of scope for changes in metabolic efficiency either upward or downward from "normal" values. First, there are several different pathways for the metabolism of energy; it is logically possible that, under energy stress, the body might switch toward more efficient pathways. Waterlow (1989) points to three possible "methods of economizing ATP [adenosine triphosphate], the unit of currency for energy exchanges": "a decrease in . . . protein turnover and ion transport across the cell membranes," of which the latter is reduced in underfeed-ing, with "some loss of the capacity for metabolic control [as a] cost of [the] adaptive process"; "reducing the amount of energy [required for a given] ATP function"; and "more efficient use of ATP for driving [given] chemical reactions," notably a switch from fast-twitch to slow-twitch muscle fibers. Pongpaew et al. (1988, 1213), comparing mildly under-nourished and (age-matched) normal Thai preschoolers, find direct chemical evidence that, for the latter, "muscle catabolism is influenced to adjust . . . protein [or] energy requirements [or both] to intake by slowing down the metabolic rate"; since these not very dissimilar groups, in a country with little within-subgroup endogamy, are almost certainly drawn from the same population, intraindividual rather than inherited adaptation is suggested.

Second, although many experiments on animals have shown that body weight cannot be maintained unless energy intake is sustained at some 40 percent above RMR, this additional amount cannot all be accounted for in terms of muscle tone or minimum obligatory physical activity (Milligan and Summers 1986). Third, RMR (even under the standard fasting and resting conditions) cannot be taken as a fixed and irreducible minimum, since RMR rates as normally measured are up to 60 percent higher than those that can be obtained with subjects under anesthesia or with sensory deprivation (Girardier and Stock 1983). Of course, the mere fact that only 40 percent of the energy cost of mainte-nance can be accounted for does not prove that increased efficiency of energy use for this purpose must be a significant part of a strain-avoiding adjustment to dietary energy stress—for example, to reduced food supply—only that it could be.

There is, moreover, evidence that some, perhaps typical, people can adapt BMR or RMR per kilogram downward under stress and that, as compared with unstressed controls, this often exceeds the 2-4 percent of intraindividual variation. Shetty (1984, 446) found that RMR per unit of surface area was 16 percent lower in undernourished, moderately active, fit, and healthy unskilled Indian laborers than in well-nourished controls, and per unit of body weight was 14 percent lower. He concluded that, apart from decreased body weight, adjustments in physical activity and possibly increased metabolic efficiency in energy utilization all contributed to maintenance of energy balance. Among poor northern Nigerian farmers, BMR per kilogram was found by Nicol and Phillips (1976), to be about 10 percent less than for well-fed Western controls. They described this as indicative of greater efficiency of energy utilization.

The problem, as with other examples of a similar kind, is how to determine whether this is *intra*personal variation, in which people have adjusted BMR per kilogram downward in response to energy stress, or *inter*personal variation in BMR per kilogram as between persons in two groups, for example, due to genetic selection (for energy-saving) among successive generations of the usually stressed group, such as Nigerian farmers in the above example. In general, however, even interpersonal variations may indicate very long-run adaptation of BMR to energy stress. That is, inter*group* differences in BMR suggest genetic adaptation to greater risks of food deprivation (or perhaps to something else), specifically in hot environments.

Thus McNeill et al. (1987) found BMR in South Indian male farm workers to be 12.1 percent below levels predicted by "world" indicators (WHO/UNU/FAO). In a scanning of data rigorously screened for reliability, Henry and Rees (1989, 154) found that for persons aged 18-60 years—usually one-sex subgroups in narrower age-bands—"all the South Asian groups, that is, Filipino, Indian, Japanese, Chinese, Malay, and Javanese" (and also Brazilians, though not groups in Yucatan or Singapore) showed average BMR per kilogram from 5 percent to 13 percent below the expected value derived from worldwide regressions of BMR per kilogram upon weight. Rural (or high-altitude) tropical groups that, exceptionally, do not show more "economical" BMR per kilogram than Westerners of similar weight, sometimes instead show significantly lower energy cost per kilogram for a given level of activity above BMR (Strickland and Ulijaszek 1990); that too may be adaptive, though it is important to heed warnings against constructing or irrefutably "adapting" stories that portray any apparently convenient outcome as an adaptation (Gould and Lewontin 1979, esp. 586-587).

How do some small-sized, hard-working people come to have BMR per kilogram of total body weight 5-13 percent lower than that typical of Western populations? Any explanation requires either that this group's BMR per kilogram of all specific organs and tissues must be similarly lower, or that they have lower body proportions of organs and tissues with high—as compared with low—metabolic rates. The latter explanation is perhaps less probable in view of the rather large changes that would be needed to account for the difference, particularly since poor Asian populations also typically have much lower fat-lean ratios. So perhaps BMR per kilogram of specific tissues has adjusted significantly downward among these populations? Many of the subpopulations of the very poor, such as Indian laboring castes, have been both energy-stressed and endogamous for many generations. More research is needed to establish whether these adjustments in BMR per kilogram are the result of natural selection among successive generations exposed to energy stress,[16] or (as in the "Sukhatme hypothesis") to intraindividual adaptation to specific periods of increased stress.

Edmundson (1979) argued the latter: that higher levels of metabolic efficiency enabled Javanese workers on a lower-energy diet to produce more work per unit than individuals with relatively higher intake. However, his findings are widely questioned. The average BMR per kilogram of his high-energy group was twice that of the low-energy group. These are quite astonishingly large variations, and no one else has produced comparable results. Interindividual variation of BMR per kilogram approaching 10 percent within a local population of similar origins and styles of life and work—a range considered reasonable by J. C. Waterlow (pers. comm.)—has been suggested by other measurements in Guatemala (Stein, Johnston, and Greinev 1988). Seasonal fluctuations in BMR per kilogram, however, appear to be considerably lower (2-4 percent), and even these are not always observed (Ferro-Luzzi, Pastore, and Sette, 1988, 37; Neumann et al. 1989, 421, for Kenya).

Edmundson's high-intake subjects also expended significantly more energy than did controls in performing standard work tasks. He concluded (Edmundson 1979) that the low energy intakes recorded (in East Java) may be related to long-term genetic adaptation and short-term phenotypic adaptation, with a decrease in BMR playing the major role in enabling a higher level of metabolic efficiency for the energy-stressed subjects. Most specialists (J. C. Waterlow, pers. comm., also citing Ferro-Luzzi) question not the role, but the size (and hence the validity of Edmundson's measurements) of variations in BMR per kilogram, and thus of the upper bound for genetic adaptation in it.

Is this adaptation of BMR per kilogram, such as it is, genetic or environmental, controllable, relevant to policy? Comparisons between dizygotic and monozygotic human twins show that (given age and sex) only about 40 percent of interpersonal variance in a person's average RMR per unit of fat-free mass is heritable (genetic) under normal circumstances (Bouchard et al. 1989). It is almost certain that some further, intrapersonal capacity to adjust RMR per kilogram in response to energy stress exists within many populations, but is much smaller than long-run adaptive differences in RMR per kilogram among populations (Edmundson and Sukhatme 1990, 271-274).

How could one detect that a person has adapted to energy stress by reducing BMR per kilogram? In practice, if an individual is preserving

---

[16]This would probably appear as lower average requirements in persons from those groups or nations that over many generations had been exposed to substantially higher levels of dietary energy stress. Three groups of eight European, seven Asiatic, and nine African students at London University were carefully matched for age, height, weight, and lean body mass. Energy costs of sitting, standing, and lying were, respectively, 13-16 percent, 10-13 percent, and 17-20 percent higher in European subjects; not significantly different between Asian and African subjects; and had very low within-group (as opposed to intergroup) variances (Geissler and Aldouri 1985, 294-296). The authors point out that the students had diets unrestricted either by class of income or by weight-loss regimes, and hypothesize that genetic differences in RMR are partly responsible.

body weight and composition despite a level of energy expenditure (assessed on the basis of that individual's previous work performance) that appears to be greater than energy intake, there are three possible explanatory factors that are hard to separate from one another. The first, which was referred to earlier, is metabolic adaptation, that is, a possible decline in RMR per kilogram of specific tissues: in effect, a reduction of unit maintenance costs. The second is increased overall efficiency of conversion or utilization of dietary energy. The third is improvement in a particular aspect of conversion efficiency, which is conveniently considered separately, namely thermogenesis: reduction in energy "wasted" through heat production.

Some scope for each of these three adjustments has been demonstrated, that is, both inter- and intraindividual variations have been demonstrated in the field and in laboratory conditions. So why is adjustment of conversion efficiency,[17] including but not limited to BMR, not a more prominent feature of scientific analyses of actual regulation and adjustment to energy stress? This is due in part to the huge difficulties and errors of measurement of intraindividual variation in free-living populations; in part to the prominence in the adjustment debate of one highly controversial and as yet not adequately supported hypothesis, that of stochastic homeostasis (Sukhatme and Margen 1982); but above all to the fact that in survival terms the double strategy of mobilizing fat reserves, thus at the same time paying off immediate energy debts and reducing future overheads, is a powerful one and for the most part—in combination with the behavioral responses (notably work adaptations) reviewed in Chapter 6 under "Ergonomic Adjustment" and except in famine—probably suffices. For metabolic efficiency of either maintenance or task-specific activities to be pressured to rise significantly (assuming that it can do so), persons in energy stress need (1) not to mobilize fat reserves, and (2) to decide to maintain task levels, structures, and ergonomics—an unlikely joint event. Moreover, to the extent that conversion efficiency does increase, for example through metabolic adjustment, there is little or no evidence about the presence or absence of adverse effects.[18]

---

[17] Such adjustment might also take the form of reduction of metabolic requirements of work over and above RMR. A WHO/Nestlé workshop of the International Dietary Energy Consultancy Group now advises defining grades 1 and 2 chronic energy deficiency as "a ratio of energy turnover to predicted BMR of less than 1.4" together with a BMI of, respectively, 17.0-18.4 and 16.0-16.9; grade 3 has BMI of less than 16.0 (irrespective of energy turnover or BMR) (Nestlé Foundation 1988, 18).

[18] An extreme possibility is that very high early death rates—almost 50 percent before age five years in The Gambia—are required for "selection of infants capable of metabolic adaptation" (Dunn Nutrition Unit 1986, 24). In other words, that there are harmful recessives, perhaps on several genes, that when expressed (that is, inherited from both parents) lead to inability to lower RMR in energy stress, and that such inability is frequently fatal in early childhood. Such sequences would also be an extreme case of the unacceptability of a process of adaptation, even though it produced an acceptable adult state for those who survived it.

There is, however, some evidence for intrapersonal adaptation via the increase of some form of conversion efficiency in response to energy stress. Infants of both sexes do appear to adjust both RMR and post-prandial heat production (specific dynamic action) upward as energy becomes more abundant (Brooke 1986, 12). Prentice and his colleagues (Nestlé Foundation 1987) provide evidence that women, even apart from pregnancy and lactation (examined separately below), have substantial powers of adjustment. It is not yet known, however, whether this is by lowering RMR (that is, reducing maintenance costs), by reducing thermogenesis (that is, by limiting additional heat loss consequent on environmental stimuli), or by increasing the efficiency of food energy conversion. In any event, women seem to have some leeway in meeting stress without reducing activity or losing body weight.

McNeill and Payne 1985 provide evidence that this capacity to "save" energy in stress is substantially more evident in women than in men. "Seasonal patterns of [low] energy intake and [high] physical activity were more marked in women, but there were not significant seasonal differences in body weight or body fat content." It makes very good sense in biological terms for females to have specialized in these kinds of energy-conserving responses, especially since investment of energy in offspring, by direct transfer, is the obvious major feature of female reproductive strategy. Investment of energy by males, on the other hand, is in the first place indirect, through food provided to the mother, and is often conditional on other circumstances, since food acquisition is usually part of a broader set of general collaborative social activities. Biological function tends to define the range and effectiveness of options for adaptive response. Thus it makes good sense if women, with the constraints imposed by reproduction, have greater capacity than men for biological adjustments that allow diversion of energy into the products of conception without varying body size, composition, or activity, while men, with a broader scope for seasonal or other short-term behavioral adaptations in activity, with or without changes in body stores, show less ability to make metabolic adjustments.

However, if women can adjust conversion efficiency by whatever means—and if a substantial part of intrapersonal capacity to adjust (as is the case for about 40 percent of interpersonal RMR per kilogram variations) is genetic—then it is doubtful that adult men have no such inherited capacity. It is not quite impossible (some genes are recessive in one sex but dominant in the other), but it is very unlikely, particularly because capacity for such adjustment is probably determined by many genes, plus environment. The extent and duration of such a capacity—which it may or may not be correct to model as its "homeostatic range" (Sukhatme and Edmundson 1989, 527)—and the causes for its variation are unknown and important for all age- and sex-groups exposed to energy stress.

If metabolic adjustment occurs and is of more than trivial magnitude, why is it so difficult to demonstrate by direct observation? The major reason is that, if habitual intake is reduced in experimental subjects, the result is always an integrated response in which changes of body weight, composition, and physical activity all play a part as well as some of the thermogenic effects discussed in the following section. In fact, several trials involving underfeeding of volunteers have been mounted during the past 60 years. In most of these, BMR per kilogram of body weight was substantially reduced. One problem in interpreting these reductions, however, lies in the uncertainty about how to correct the results for the accompanying changes in weight and fat content. There are regression equations that can be used to make corrections for the differences in whole-body BMR between normal individuals of different body sizes as well as to adjust for differences of ethnicity, climate, age, and sex. However, when these equations are used to correct for the effect of low body weight on BMR in free-living under-nourished subjects, or of weight loss on BMR in experimentally under-fed subjects, they generally do not account for the whole of the decline. The question is, Can that unaccountable component be attributed to metabolic adaptation and, if so, could victims of energy stress in field conditions (in some cases) avail themselves of it?

The measurements by Shetty (1984) of low BMR values in poor Indian agricultural laborers have already been mentioned. These were considerably below those of a control group. Part of this, but only part, can be discounted on the grounds that the controls had untypically high values (McNeill 1986). However, the poor laborers had endured a period of unemployment and had BMI values as low as 16.6. This precludes any direct comparison of BMR with controls of substantially higher BMI unless one has recourse to mathematical corrections for height, weight, or "surface area"; but which, if any, of the many equations derived from data on "normal" subjects of different body sizes is valid for this?

In experimental studies, the discrepancies between observed and predicted metabolic rates are also considerable. For example, the study most often quoted is a semistarvation trial reported by Keys et al. (1950). Thirty-two men were given half their normal energy intake for 24 weeks and lost an average 24 percent of their initial body weight. The BMRs fell by an average of 39 percent, although the amount of lean tissue loss would have led to a predicted reduction in BMR of only 22 percent. This would leave a possible 17 percent to be counted as metabolic adjustment. There are still some problems of interpretation; there were major changes in body composition, and the subjects were not equilibrated at their reduced weights but were almost immediately placed on a recovery regime.

However, the decline in BMR in these experiments was progressive throughout the 24 weeks, and by 8 weeks was already greater than could be accounted for by the change in weight. It seems to be generally accepted that this experiment did demonstrate a real response of BMR per kilogram to underfeeding, and that this was probably not a result only of weight or composition changes. However, it is not widely ac-cepted as evidence of the existence of metabolic adaptation as a general phenomenon. The argument is that these subjects were studied during the process of semistarvation and could not be regarded as having made a sustainable adjustment to the stress to which they were exposed. They had lost a considerable amount of weight and their physical activity had fallen to a very low level before any real (that is, unaccounted for in terms of size or composition changes) effect on BMR could be measured.

The problem is that with the measurement techniques available, it is difficult to distinguish such real changes in BMR when smaller levels of stress or shorter exposure times are used.

A study by Benedict et al. (1919) has received less attention but is more relevant to metabolic adaptation under conditions of moderate stress. Twelve men were subjected to a 10 percent reduction in body weight (a change of BMI from 22.8 down to 20.0) by a careful adjustment of each individual's energy intake, which amounted on average to a 30 percent reduction. Their weights were stabilized at the lower level and maintained for three months. The subjects were urged to maintain, as far as they could, their habitual patterns of physical activity during both work and recreation. Detailed studies were made of changes of physiological and psychological function including, for example, the energy cost of a 10-kilometer walk before and after weight reduction. In these subjects there was a decline in BMR of 12 percent greater than could be accounted for on the basis of body weight change. The energy cost of walking, however, was reduced simply in direct proportion to the weight loss; BMR efficiency rose, but task efficiency, metabolic or ergonomic, was unaltered. Still, since BMR accounts for 60-70 percent of typical energy expenditure even in hard-working farm laborers, a 12 percent cut (with a weight reduction of 10 percent) would still leave a reduction of about 8 percent in dietary energy requirements over and above the reduction due to weight loss. Such resistance to strain would substantially add to the already large energy-saving effects of smallness, spelled out in Table 2, and would strengthen the case for seeing smallness as adaptive. Of course, this interaction tells nothing about the acceptability or otherwise of smallness, lower BMR per kilogram, or their interaction; but it is, at least, not obvious why the last two forms of energy economy have any costs at all. In any case, the onus of proof appears to lie with those who assert that such costs exist.

Garby (1987) has used a different method for analyzing the effects on BMR of both over- and underfeeding. He calculates the changes in BMR that would be expected from the gains or losses of fat and lean tissue, that is, assuming constant values for the metabolic rates per kilogram of fat and lean tissue, which he derived from independent studies. Garby finds that three studies on overconsumption show an average excess of 5 percent (range of 3-7 percent) of BMR unaccounted for by change of weight; eight underfeeding trials found an average shortfall of 7.5 percent (range of 0-17 percent) of BMR below the predicted values. If the latter range is replicated in larger trials, the importance for Third World nutrition policy is very great. It should be noted however, that there are no comparable data for children. Nor is it known whether BMR adaptation is less or more when the sources of energy stress are (say) heavier work or infection rather than underfeeding, or when they are briefer or longer.

The last of the three possible explanations for reduced BMR per kilogram under energy stress is that there could be a reduction in the amounts of extra heat normally produced as a side effect of adjustments to some other kinds of environmental stresses such as infections, cold exposure, emotional stresses. The measurement problems of distinguishing this from metabolic or food efficiency changes under field conditions would be insuperable. One can, however, look to laboratory trials for an assessment of the possible magnitude of the energy saving that might result.

Adjustment of Thermogenesis

In this context, thermogenesis means heat production above the level associated with normal metabolism in a resting, fasted, and thermoneutral state. Such additional heat can arise in response to a number of stimuli (usually short-term), the most important of which for this discussion are (1) exposure to cold;[19] (2) hormones such as adrenaline or norepinephrine; (3) emotional stress such as anger or fear, which is partly mediated by (2); (4) ingestion of food, with or without exercise; and (5) toxins, notably those generated by infectious disease processes.

It is possible that a reduction in the amount of heat produced in response to any or all of the above stimuli might be an effective way to respond to energy stress arising from a source other than those. If so, are the costs of such a reduction likely to be acceptable? In general there are three aspects to consider: the maximum extent to which metabolic rate can be increased in response to a stimulus, and hence the potential for saving energy by reducing such a response; the likely frequency of such stimuli; and, when these are transient (for example, meals, short bursts of physical activity, episodes of anger, fear, and so forth), the length of time over which appreciable levels of metabolic response persist after the stimulus is removed.

Responses to Cold

Cold exposure can result in two different biological mechanisms for thermogenesis. Shivering involves involuntary muscular work. Nonshivering thermogenesis (NST) involves direct generation of heat by an increase in metabolic rate.

In the earlier discussion of low environmental temperature as a source of stress (Chapter 4, under "Temperature"), one example of adjustment was described: the !Kung's ability to lower RMR and skin and core temperatures to reduce body heat losses, and thus to obviate the need to use up energy for the shivering response. Since they also have lowered resting metabolic rate throughout sleeping, it can be assumed that they also suppress the nonshivering response to cold, thereby reducing their overall maintenance requirements. Such suppression of the need for thermogenesis could also be a means of repartitioning stress from a source such as dietary constraint, or an uncompensated increase in daytime workload. However, this is the only example found. Responses to temperature stress per se usually take the form of avoidance—lowering the threshold temperature for thermal neutrality by

---

[19]In this case, specifically excluding effects due to shivering, that is, to involuntary muscular work.

increased clothing or sheltering, or raising environmental temperature by heating. In permanently warm climates, moreover, or if clothing and shelter are sufficient to ensure that no stimulus to NST occurs, reduction of the potential capacity for making such responses would obviously confer no benefit.

Effects of Hormones

A common experimental technique for studying thermogenesis is to give small doses of the hormones noradrenaline or norepinephrine by injection to human subjects and measure the increase in RMR that results. It has been argued that the magnitude of these increments is a measure of the general capacity of an individual to make a thermogenic response (that is, independently of the nature of the stimulus).

This technique gives responses that in terms of maximum increment of oxygen uptake are quite large even for some "chronically undernourished, but physically active and otherwise healthy" groups. Shetty et al. (1987) compared such men, aged 19-28, with two other groups—one matched for height and age but of normal weight, the other underweight for their height but not undernourished (that is, they were constitutionally thin)—for response to norepinephrine stimuli repeated at five-minute intervals. Shorter, lighter men (that is, those classified as chronically undernourished) showed 40-45 percent lower NST responses to the first two such stimuli than the underweight controls, despite the fact that these had similar body mass indices and fat-free body mass. The differences declined as the two stimuli (doses of norepinephrine) were increased in size, but subsequently increased and stabilized at a high level (over 40 percent) as the number of stimuli, of moderate size, was increased from 2 to 12 doses (at five-minute intervals).

Plainly, NST response to norepinephrine is sharply lower—at least for small or moderate stimuli, or for frequently repeated or long-duration stimuli—among people in energy stress. As is often the case, it cannot be determined whether this represents durable (perhaps genetic) adjustment in some people to *prolonged* stress, or adjustments that most or all persons make in *periods* of stress. In either case, though the total amount of NST is not large (typically only 10-12 percent of intake at energy balance for a healthy adult), a 40-45 percent saving of this would be a significant resistance to strain, and hence an apparently adaptive adjustment to energy stress—if one can infer that this capacity of (some) undernourished persons to reduce NST after norepinephrine stimuli also exists for other stimuli.

Indeed, Shetty et al. (1987) conjecture that NST responses to injected norepinephrine can be regarded as a measure of capacity to respond to cold. They believe that their findings largely explain why undernourished people suffer higher rates of death and damage due to cold exposure. If this is so, energy saving by reduced NST would not normally be adaptive, let alone acceptable, as a way to counter energy stress in (say) the hills of Nepal or other cold places. In warm places—the habitats of the vast majority of persons at risk of energy stress—curtailment of NST under cold stress might not carry any penalty but would happen much too seldom to result in significant energy saving.

Emotional Stress

If, in addition to being a measure of capacity to respond to cold, NST response to norepinephrine is also an index of emotional stress reactions, then an overall reduction in NST responsiveness as a means of saving energy might have adverse implications. For example, capacity for arousal and effective response to sudden hazards, threats, and so forth, might be reduced as a consequence. However, calmer and less-energy-using responses to many situations—from minor irritations through family quarrels to serious hazards requiring measured response rather than "fight or flight"—could even be a desirable result of adaptation to energy stress.

Diet-induced Thermogenesis

A distinction was made earlier between diet-induced thermogenesis and specific dynamic action. Specific dynamic action accounts for part of the heat released as a result of the ingestion of food. The metabolic processes for transferring the energy that is stored in chemical bonds in food constituents, proteins, fats, and carbohydrates to the processes of synthesis of body constituents are less than 100 percent efficient: waste heat is therefore produced as an inevitable result. It is most likely that this is simply an obligatory loss and is in fixed proportion to the quantity of nutrients metabolized. However, since quite large amounts of energy are involved, it is reasonable to ask whether an increase in efficiency of energy coupling might be a conceivable response to energy stress. There is as yet no answer to this except to say that any alternative metabolic pathways that would result in greater energetic efficiency would almost certainly have already been selected for as part of the evolutionary process, unless there was some serious offsetting disadvantage.

Diet-induced thermogenesis, on the other hand, is a response of the body to the stimulus of eating and is similar in nature to the effects of hormones. Since diet-induced thermogenesis depends not only on the size, frequency, and composition of meals (that is, the size and frequency of the stimulus) but also on the physiological response of the body, its reduction might be a possible energy-saving adjustment to stress. This could be mediated by behavioral factors, most obviously by reduced numbers of snacks or concentration of energy intake into a smaller number of meals or both (Prentice et al. 1983b). There is also evidence of physiological reduction in diet-induced thermogenesis as a response resulting from energy stress (Waterlow 1989, 21-22; Blaxter and Waterlow 1985, 148; Grande 1984, 15). It is not clear how much of this is contingent upon prior depletion of body reserves; a strong link is suggested by the evidence (Ashworth and Millward 1986, 161) that children in need of catch-up growth, given the same meal, show smaller postprandial increases in RMR when weight gain in the preceding period has been less.

Clearly some reduction in diet-induced thermogenesis is automatic if, but only if, energy stress is caused by reduced intake. In addition, diet-induced thermogenesis is related to (some, for example Miller

[1982], say it potentiates) the long-term effects of exercise. A short burst of physical activity not only has to be paid for in proportion to the work done but also acts as a stimulus, much like diet-induced thermogenesis, in causing thermogenesis above the normal resting rate for some hours afterward. There is evidence that, when diet-induced thermogenesis and exercise occur together, the effect on heat production is more than simply additive. However, the magnitude of energy cost due to the joint effects of eating and exercise, while extended over time, is still relatively small, amounting to only one-fifth to one-quarter of the whole of the extra heat production stimulated by eating—that is, 2-3 percent out of the total 10-12 percent of the maintenance energy needs of normal subjects that is counted as diet-induced thermogenesis (James 1985). Hence, if chronic undernutrition leads to a 60 percent reduction in these two responses—properly classified as resistance to stress, rather than to strain, which does not materialize—there is a maximum saving of between 1.2 and 1.8 percent of total energy requirements.

To the extent that energy stress leads to reduced intensity of effort or reduced duration of fairly intense effort, it is possible to distinguish three forms of energy saving: (1) direct energy requirements of work are reduced—resistance to strain; (2) diet-induced thermogenesis is reduced; (3) RMR per kilogram is reduced for about 12 hours after the energetic work stops. Both (2) and (3) constitute resistance to stress and are affected by genetic endowment (Poehlman and Horton 1989). This probably helps explain why some adults are more prone than others to reduce work intensity in response to energy stresses; those who do reduce it may well obtain more energy saving (absolutely, per kilogram, and per rupee's worth of food earned by work) from such a reduction than nonreducers would.

Infections

The thermogenic effects of infections can be quite considerable, ranging from 10 to 15 percent increase in RMR for every 1°C rise in body temperature. The mechanisms involved are complex and constitute part of a general defense process. This ensures favorable conditions for action against invading organisms by the immune systems of the body, which work better at higher temperatures, and for the processes of breakdown and elimination of the toxic substances produced by that action (Keusch and Farthing 1986). Clearly, chronic recurrent infections, such as malaria, could significantly increase energy expenditure. Given frequent episodes of infection, an effective counter to additional energy stress might be a general reduction in the size of the febrile response.

Would there be countervailing disadvantages? In the present state of knowledge, this is hard to say. Partly, this is because infectious episodes are in any case almost always accompanied by depression of appetite. It has been suggested (Tomkins and Watson 1989) that this is part of a biological "infection control strategy," the effect of which paradoxically is to reduce the danger of "thermal runaway." The risk of excessive (sometimes fatal) rises in body temperature can be reduced by cutting down the intake of iron and other substances that catalyze the thermogenic reactions. It seems, therefore, that while thermogenesis is a necessary part of defense against infections, there is a fine balance between adequate and excessive responses. Up to a point, some concession to the proverbial advice to "starve a fever" might make some sense; conversely, some reduction in febrile response might be an effective adaptation, not only via (partial) avoidance of energy stress due to infection but conceivably also via improved prospects of recovery from it.

Adjustments to Stress During Reproduction: Pregnancy, Lactation, and Birth Frequency

A long-run avoidance of source of nutritional stress in girls—lowering reproductive efficiency and therefore not likely to be adaptive in the Darwinian sense but certainly acceptable for those who believe that large families place a severe, often unwanted, burden on women, on the poor, and on the economic growth process—can be seen in delayed menarche and earlier menopause (Eveleth 1985, 34). A more short-run response of the same type is increased length of postpartum amenorrhea. Furthermore, ovulation is thought not to occur if fat reserves fall below a certain critical threshold. The mechanism is thought to maximize the probability that a given pregnancy will succeed, that is, to minimize energy investment per successful birth. Ovulation is prevented only while an infant is dependent on the mother (Quandt 1984).

Under famine conditions, it is probable that poor nutrition will also depress fertility, delay menarche, and decrease the period of fecundity (Dirks 1980). Variations in hormonal levels among the women of the Kalahari are thought to decrease fertility during food shortages.

Bentley (1985) has pointed to a correlation between the season of least energy expenditure and a higher rate of conception among the !Kung San. Unusually long weaning periods may also contribute to the long birth interval. Conceptions among this group are high when intakes are highest and body weight at a maximum (July-August). Analysis of data in Taiwan also suggests links between conception and seasonality in diet (Mosher 1979), as do careful data from Bangladesh (Chambers, Longhurst, and Pacey 1981, 150-152).

The balance of evidence from Bangladesh and several other countries suggests that birth cycles—and, by implication, successful conception—are "timed" so as to reduce quite substantially (below the expected value of about 50 percent) the proportion of all infants born, who reach ages of between 7 and 12 months, during the second half of the main wet season. This remarkable adaptation, which might of course be partly explained by either cultural or inherited behavioral patterns, reduces the risk of overlap between the time when the child is (1) likeliest to receive reduced care because of the pressures of farmwork, and (2) in transition, having lost inborn and maternally transmitted (passive) immunity but not yet acquired active immunity to several infections that are major sources of energy stress (Schofield 1974).

Even if the risks to child health are reduced by thus ensuring that transition does not coincide with the greatest likelihood of household energy stress, there is no reason to believe that the resulting birth seasonality is an optimal, or even desirable, corrective to the seasonal adult energy stress cycle. In other words, better adaptation to energy stress bearing upon infants, through avoidance of the source (through timing of pregnancy and birth), might need to be set against the cost of less favorable timing for the mother. However, the recent evidence that energy requirements of pregnancy can in some circumstances be much lower than had been thought means that the amount of compensatory reduction of physical activity may also be less than expected. In such circumstances, therefore, it is probably adaptive for birth seasonality to be adjusted in the light of the prospective effects of seasonal energy stress on children rather than of the mothers' current requirements.

As well as the timing of conceptions, three other important adaptations to energy stress in pregnancy may be biological, behavioral, or a mixture. First, several studies report an overall reduction in physical activity during pregnancy (McNeill and Payne 1985). If "rest is best" for the hungry fetus (Briend 1984) this is a desirable adaptation, supported by conformity to a cultural norm. As with birth cycles, research is needed to establish whether the adaptation is biological or behavioral. This is a matter of some policy significance, since policies affecting adaptation, however unintentionally, can save—or waste—lives.

Second, more efficient utilization of body-fat stores has been observed in pregnant women. This change has also been found, and measured, for lactating women, notably in The Gambia (Rowland et al. 1981; Lawrence et al. 1987). Lactating women appear to have a raised mobility of fat stores compared with nonpregnant, nonlactating women. This increased mobility involves both greater fat deposition during the dry season and greater fat utilization during the wet season. Therefore, weight change is not an obligatory counterpart to successful lactation.[20] Prolonged lactation—so typical of rural communities in Asia and Africa—extends the period for such increased mobility of fat stores and appears to be otherwise adaptive to energy stress. For the mother, it causes body fat to decline, reducing the chance of ovulation and subsequent pregnancy. For the weanling, it probably safeguards the diet against shortage of "outside" foods. For the baby to follow, it increases spacing and thus improves child care.

Third, deposition of fat obviously tends to increase during pregnancy; one of the functions of weight gain during pregnancy is to develop energy stores for fetal growth and lactation. These stores act as a buffer in the diet; if the efficiency of storage and transfer to the fetus is total, then the effect of supplementation upon the well-being of the fetus in late pregnancy would be the same regardless of when the supplementation is given (Lechtig et al. 1975). Such perfectly adapted

---

[20]In the supplemental trials in The Gambia, it was also found that season had a similar impact on body size and energy stores during pregnancy, irrespective of the stage of pregnancy.

storage efficiency is of course not present: it is shown by Dutch famine studies (Stein and Susser 1975) and others (Viegas et al. 1982) that, below a certain threshold, negative maternal energy balance in the third trimester adversely affects birth weight even if earlier food intakes allowed the mother to build up energy stores. Also, more maternal body-store is not the main determinant of the neonate's size: "maternal anthropometric variables accounted for only between 6 percent (height and fat mass) and 20 percent (fat-free mass) of [its] total variance" in The Gambia (Lawrence, McKillop, and Durnin 1989, 59). More than maternal body mass for the fetus, breast milk can be regarded as insurance for the young child, making it relatively independent of food availability to maintain its food intake. Most unweaned children receive most nutrients from breast milk (for example, in rural Bangladesh: Brown, Black, and Becker 1982). Therefore, food ingested in seasons of plenty can be transferred to children in seasons of need.

A fourth sort of adaptation to energy stress, this time clearly biological, applies in both pregnancy and lactation and involves increased overall conversion efficiency. As discussed in the first section of this chapter, the capacity of adult men to achieve this adaptation is controversial, hard to measure (and hard to separate, as between reduced BMR per kilogram and improved efficiency in thermogenesis), and probably rather small. However, recent evidence (Nestlé Foundation 1987) from five populations—four comprising poor rural women in the tropics—suggests effective resistance to strain via increases, probably substantial, in metabolic efficiency during pregnancy. This implies that the energy requirements in pregnant women given in FAO/WHO/UNU 1985 are exaggerated and, if "implemented," could needlessly transfer food from preschoolers who require it more or map pregnant women into obesity or both. This appears to apply even more strongly in lactation: among rural Gambian women, "during the first 12 months post-partum, RMR was reduced by up to 100 kcal/day compared with conception and with late lactation (15-18 months)"; only during the first month of lactation could this be in part attributed to reduced physical activity (Lawrence and Whitehead 1989). It will be interesting to learn why pregnant and lactating women are better at reducing RMR in energy stress than others—and whether such adaptation has hidden costs.[21]

---

[21]A very important point is raised by Beaton (1989, 299-300): does the apparently acceptable adaptation reported by Prentice et al. (1983a, 1983b) conceal reductions in "discretionary activity . . . including social functions and psychosocial development," suggested by the anecdotal observation that when lactating women in The Gambia were given food supplements, they sang as they worked? Such adaptation, while less distressing to its victims than some, is surely not acceptable in the longer term. However, the case for inferring it is still speculative and depends on Beaton's doubt that "improvements in the efficiency of food absorption or of metabolism are a likely explanation" of the results of the Gambian studies on pregnant and lactating women. The reasons stated in Dunn Nutrition Unit (1986, 71-72) for placing more emphasis on such adaptive possibilities appear to be sound.

It certainly has limits. Although, in The Gambia (Prentice et al. 1983a, 1983b), dietary supplements raised mothers' energy intakes (from 1,400 to 1,800 kilocalories per woman per day) by 30-40 percent during lactation, this had no effect on the quantity of breast milk. The impact during pregnancy was a 15-25 percent rise in birth weight when births took place in the wet season, though with no effect in the dry season. Seasonal energy stress from high work levels and low food intake may therefore exhaust some of any capacity for metabolic adaptation to further stress in pregnancy.

Whether genetic-environmental interactions or changes in behavior (food mix? work timing?) alone can significantly improve adult or child efficiency of food conversion in energy stress—or can reduce the costs (whatever they may be) of any given feasible improvements in conversion efficiency—is as yet quite mysterious. That such effects may be important is suggested by evidence that the timing of food supplementation, vis-à-vis season of work-food stress, critically affects the "level of dietary energy efficiency adaptation which may be naturally switched on and off with the annual cycle of hungry and post-harvest seasons" (Diaz et al. 1989, 4). Research is needed into what, if anything, might be done, either through public policy or by actions taken by individuals or households facing energy stress, to increase their prospects for such adaptation through "dietary energy efficiency" at a given set of costs (or to lower those costs, if they are identifiable and significant). "We need a great deal more basic research on energy and protein metabolism in order to establish the possibilities for adaptation to low intakes . . . . [S]hortage of funding for [such] research . . . will . . . seriously handicap our efforts to improve the nutrition of the people of the Third World" (Waterlow 1989, 5).

6

Behavioral Responses to the Stress Environment

Three aspects of a person's work output that may be affected by dietary energy stress have been identified by Viteri et al. (1981, 279). The biological effects, that is, the physical capacity to sustain work of various types and durations, were reviewed in Chapter 5. The effects on voluntary work duration and intensity and on adult work efficiency will be considered here.

Behavioral choices, determined by external incentives as well as by psychological preferences, link the three effects. For example, if labor supply is ample, working households often respond to energy stress by spreading work over a longer period; thus they reduce energy expenditure per day, either time at work or intensity per unit of time, during stress. On the other hand, if a hard task must be done in a critical period (for example, clearing bush before the rains), while those usually working at this task are scarce yet energy-stressed, then the options are different: defer other tasks, call on reserves to swell the labor force, or accept assorted unpleasantnesses or nonenergy costs to increase ergonomic efficiency.

Workers lose weight from energy stress only to the extent that its conversion into strain cannot be avoided by some combination of increased metabolic efficiency (if feasible) and one or more of three strategies: raise biological conversion into applied effort per unit of energy ingested and expended—for example, as the muscles benefit from training effect (see the first section of Chapter 5); reduce energy expended (working time or expenditure of energy per unit of time); increase ergonomic efficiency or units of economic output per unit of applied effort.

Apart from adjustments to adults' economic (including domestic) activity, changed household behavior under energy stress can affect children's work, play, or management as well as household food acquisition or composition.

Reduced Energy Expenditure

Several studies (cited in Ferro-Luzzi 1985, 66) show that short adults, or those with low lean body mass, take longer to produce the "same" output, though a minority of studies linked to task types involving body translation rather than heavy lifting do not show this. In most tasks—not involving unusually high energy expenditures, say above 45 percent of VO_2max—this is largely or wholly a behavioral choice, not an unavoidable metabolic requirement. Slower performance of a given task uses up less energy. Is repartitioning of the source of stress, by choosing longer periods of slower (and ergonomically more efficient) work, an unacceptable adaptation? Sometimes; but there need be no substantial loss in income, production, or welfare from slower work.

First, work may be better done if it is done more slowly. In some of the tasks cited above (weeding, coffee picking), this is certainly the case, although an employee on a piece rate will usually not receive the benefits. This is reflected in the absence, in rigorous studies, of any impact of moderately smaller body size, which is associated with slower performance of some tasks, on rural wage rates (Vosti 1984).

Second, a great deal of spare time may be available. Energy stress often occurs in heavily populated regions. With the important exception of the few weeks each year of very high employment in peak farming activities, the costs of a decision to perform a task more slowly may be small.

Third, it may well be possible to "make" time for slower work on key tasks in energy stress by deferring other tasks. Cattle-care and domestic work are typically, and sensibly, "packed" into otherwise slack seasons (Hopper 1955; Lipton 1983a). This usually amounts to saying that such activities are concentrated by temporarily stressed households into less-stressed times of year, enabling critical tasks to be done without haste (that is, without specially high use of energy) during periods of potential energy stress. This means repartitioning the source of stress between high- and low-priority (or high- and low-shiftability) tasks or times.

This repartitioning has three advantages. First, behavior that keeps, say, fortnightly energy expenditure moving in parallel with fortnightly intake is a more efficient response to fluctuating intake than is deposition and storage of fat—and even more of lean—because the latter biological responses themselves use up some energy. Second, to perform the same tasks more slowly when food is short, even if this means a longer working day, on balance reduces energy expenditure (and hence avoids strain) directly because the relationships between rate of energy expenditure and load, speed of walking, and gradient are non-linear; the higher loads, speeds, and so forth, cause disproportionate increases in energy expenditure rates. Thus shorter times do not compensate for higher rates of work. The higher the body weight, the greater the "saving" from slowness (Pimental and Pandolf 1979), so that very small and light populations have rather less prospect for successful adaptations along this route. Third, however, there is an indirect saving: by smoothing out the daily amount of work done, one avoids faster work performance that raises subsequent BMR more, and for a longer period, than does gradual completion of work (Miller 1982).

Apart from working less hard, working for shorter hours could reduce energy expenditure. This latter method, however, runs counter to some of the ways in which people seek to avoid energy stress; for example, longer journeys for food-gathering or for work-seeking. Moreover, the effect of either reduction, in time worked or in energy-intensity per hour, on total energy expended is limited because voluntary activity in working adults typically accounts for only 20-25 percent of total energy expenditure when averaged over time. This means that if all of a shortfall in available food energy is compensated for by a reduction in work output, the latter may be drastically affected: reducing maintenance cost by losing weight might be a more effective strategy.

Table 3 shows the outcomes of adjusting to a 10 percent cut in food intake either by simply reducing energy expended on productive work or leisure activities, or by lowering maintenance energy needs through reduced body weight, together with a small reduction in work or leisure needs. The figures in the first column are representative of those described by McNeill (1986) for small landowners (1.25-2.50 acres) in Tamil Nadu State in India. The second column shows that to adjust to a 10 percent reduction in intake without a change either in body weight or in the energy associated with activities necessary to sustain life and health (calculated as 140 percent of BMR) would require a nearly 50 percent cut in productive work output or leisure activities or both. The third column shows the outcome of adjustment of 10 percent in productive work or leisure, together with a reduced body weight (and hence lowered maintenance because of lower BMR). This might seem a somewhat desperate strategy. However, the figures in the third column correspond quite closely with those observed by McNeill for landless workers in the same village, who did in fact have food energy intakes on average 10 percent lower than the small landowners (together with BMIs of around 18-19) despite maintaining very similar expenditure rates at work. In addition to the savings directly linked to reduced body weight, further adjustments are likely. Reducing the rate of expenditure during productive work might improve the efficiency of work output (see "Ergonomic Adjustment" section below). Longer time spent working at a lower rate might be at the expense of time and energy spent on leisure activities. Overall, these adjustments might imply no loss of production despite the reduced expenditure on work and leisure activities.

Table 3—Reduced energy expenditure or body weight?

| | | Intake Reduced by 10 Percent | |
Item	Initial State	Reduced Productive Work	Reduced Body Weight
Energy intake (kilocalories/day)	2,600	2,340	2,340
Maintenance energy (1.4 x BMR: kilocalories/day)[a]	2,000	2,000	1,740
Energy cost of productive work and leisure (kilocalories/day)	600	340	550
Body weight (kilograms)	55.0	55.0	48.0
Body mass index[b]	21.0	21.0	18.1

[a]BMR is basal metabolic rate.
[b]Weight in kilograms divided by the square of height in meters.

In general, there appears to be justification for Ferro-Luzzi's (1985, 63) doubts about the assumption that most "long-term adaptation to low energy intake may be achieved by means of curtailing physical activity," especially for "poor people who mostly depend on their own physical labor for survival." Still, even a small saving in energy expended is worth having, especially as one of many low-cost responses to stress. It should be noted that such savings in energy expenditure are behavioral responses to one or several of a wide range of impairments of working capacity: by infections, by energy stress, and by anemia, which decreases the blood's capacity to transport oxygen (Spurr 1984). Anemia and some infections are synergistic with undernutrition but can occur separately.

Who is able to reduce work, and thereby repartition some of these combined sources of stress? People with several sources of command over food, especially if they have different energy requirements, can adjust to energy stress by sacrificing some of their normal variety in food and work jointly. This is especially notable among pastoralists. The Senegalese Ferlo, in the higher-stress rainy season, offset food shortage by less energy-using recourse to food gathered in the wild. On the other hand, Ota and Twa women in equatorial forests in Zaire reduce their activity in the hungry season by ceasing to gather and scoop fish in the forest while manioc fields are being planted. At the end of the wet season, heavy physical work is carried out (Pagezy 1984). In periods of stress the Tlokwa in the Eastern Kalahari reduce their energy expenditure in obtaining food by adjusting the balance of agriculture—horticulture, animal husbandry, and hunting-gathering (Grivetti 1978).

Behavioral specialization often records "fossilized," learned changes by different groups in achieving avoidance or repartitioning responses to various sources of energy stress. This is exemplified by sexual specialization. The women of the Ache of Paraguay (Hurtado et al. 1985) acquire 13 percent of total calories produced by the foraging group but 80 percent of the total vegetable calories; the men exploit resources with high energy content per kilogram, such as honey and game. It is hypothesized that women exploit the less energy-dense resources because these are more compatible with their carrying and acquiring duties, while men's tasks require more energy-dense foods to permit stalking of mobile animal resources.

Activity specializations are both cause and effect of evolved anthropometry, in part as joint ways to repartition sources of potential stress so as to reduce actual stress for each specializing person. Thus, different activity patterns between lowlanders and highlanders in Papua New Guinea are related to differences in body mass in those groups (Ohtsuka et al. 1985). Northern and inland people are thinner, while riverine and coastal people are fatter; the former travel on foot and over longer distances, especially for sago-working and hunting. They also carry heavy items such as raw sago flour, garden crops, and firewood. The riverine and coastal people work in places near the village and use river canoes to transport their goods.

Specialization in tasks has been noted in studies of the marginally malnourished. School-aged Colombian boys with low weight-for-height specialize in tasks that involve translation or lifting of the body, which could be achieved with less O_2 consumption, since less total work is involved due to their diminished body mass (Barac-Nieto, Spurr, and Reina 1984). This seems to be a clear case of adaptive, learned response, partitioning the sources of potential stress so as to minimize realized stress on the most vulnerable. Whether the adaptation is acceptable depends on the effect on the income, well-being, and prospects of both groups, especially the marginally malnourished, but also on the effect of alternative ways to respond. With energy stress, as with balance-of-payments deficits, any "structural adjustment" cannot be praised or damned without reviewing the effects of the alternatives, including nonadjustment.

Types of task coupled with work intensity are important types of adaptation. In their studies of pregnant women, Lawrence et al. (1985) found that pregnancy alters the intensity (and hence energy expenditure) of some tasks such as bending and digging, but not of others such as walking, standing, or pounding. Pregnant women may adapt toward more nonloadbearing activities, avoiding intensive use of arm and back muscles.

Ergonomic Adjustment

As discussed above, households seek low-cost responses to energy stress by adjusting task intensity, duration, timing, selection, and allocation among household members. However, some tasks must be done by a particular individual within a particular period, whether he or she is malnourished or not. Those who are malnourished may then seek a way of performing these tasks that minimizes the energy costs, thereby avoiding the source of stress, or else accepting it but adapting behavior so as to tolerate low-level strain. The following is a list of behaviors that might help.

1. As mentioned earlier in the discussion of work capacity, "training effects" result in reduced energy costs. Slowly increasing periods of physically intense work gradually increase muscular efficiency and aerobic capacity. This reduces the energy cost of performing those tasks. Of course, there is an initial fixed cost of training and working at high physical intensity. Especially in nonstressed periods, persons prone to stress can engage in task specialization to develop the training effect for particular muscles as well as for the heart-lung system. These then operate more efficiently in the stressed period, reducing energy cost and hence stress.

2. Task specialization is a viable strategy. Certain individuals, due to their physiological characteristics or their aerobic training, expend less energy at a given task. The worldwide tendency for men to clear land and plow, and for women to transplant rice and weed, is almost certainly related to the muscular efficiency of each sex. If so, the proper feminist critique may well be of the relative rewards and prestige attached to these tasks, not of gender specialization in them. Specialization in tasks among the marginally malnourished can be a way of reducing activity, but it can also form part of a strategy leading to greater ergonomic efficiency.

3. Physiological factors operate in such a way that the energy costs of performing tasks can be reduced either by slowing the speed of performance or by spreading out reduced work loads over longer times. Examples of this have already been mentioned. Pimental and Pandolf (1979) show that the effects of load (weight carried) and grade (steepness of slope) on expenditure rate are both nonlinear, so that there are trade-offs to be made between total cost of transporting a load and the time required.

4. Even identical twins of the same sex and body mass, required to perform the same task during an exactly given time, would in all likelihood act differently if only one were energy-stressed. Many choices of use exist for almost every voluntary muscle in performing a given function. In particular, there is almost always a trade-off between comfort and energy-saving. The classic "fat man's reaction"—picking up objects with a long stretch, or even with bare feet instead of hands, to avoid getting up and walking—reflects (and helps to cause) his fatness and the associated high energy costs of body translation. Under energy stress, such reactions can be adopted, and reactions that "waste" calories to gain comfort can be avoided. These options extend beyond standard ergonomic choices. Among dispensable, energy-costly, but comfort-increasing behaviors are such things as fidgeting, scratching, wiping away sweat, or more frequent interruptions of work.

Of course, it is not acceptable that people should be denied reasonable comfort because they are poor. The point, however, is to identify poor people's least damaging responses to a situation in which some damage is inevitable. More efficient, but less pleasant, work may be a preferable alternative to more serious strains resulting from dietary energy stress.

The standard journals and books on ergonomics appear to have little to say about work-method responses—successful, adaptive, or otherwise—to energy stress. Such responses, quite apart from changes in working time or intensity, could be important, however.

Children: Activity, Play, Management, Learning

Torún and Viteri (1981) found that preschool children reduce activity in response to reduced energy intake. They suggested that reduced activity is the initial response of preschool children, followed by reduced weight gain. Graham et al. (1981, 551) also argue that since "over 70 percent of energy intake for children is used for maintenance, a variable but significant proportion for activity, and only a small proportion for growth . . . when [energy intake is] marginally inadequate, growth and weight gain may be curtailed, but activity is more likely to be sacrificed to maintain some growth."

Is this sacrifice acceptable or are there significant costs? It is doubtful whether this reduced play does lasting damage except in severe or prolonged undernutrition or where it—or the reduced growth—is a marker for likely continued exposure to deprivation. A study in the

Indian Punjab (Kielmann et al. 1978, 3-27) concludes that "nutritional deficiency in the range commonly encountered in a rural ambulatory community seemed not to be associated with permanent psychomotor impairment." Reduced play, however, obviously means a loss in happiness—in utility even if not in capability.

It also remains possible that poor children in primary school are impaired in socializing or in school performance by undernutrition. Certainly that is so for those seriously affected. For mild or moderate stunting on its own, however, there is no evidence of lasting damage to school performance (see the section on "Cognition" in Chapter 5). Socializing may nevertheless be impaired by lower height or temporarily worse school performance. Yet for policy purposes the question remains whether "food first" is a sensible approach, for these somewhat stunted children, to problems of social status whose underlying cause is created by their families' lack of land, markets, or politico-economic power.

Spurr et al. (1986), Spurr (1987), and Desai et al. (1984) found that adolescents were unlike preschoolers in their response to undernutrition: they tended to reduce growth via biological response rather than play via behavioral response. Peer pressure minimized the effect of malnutrition on activity levels in adolescents. They were able to perform at activity levels similar to their peers, in part because of the lower energy cost of maintaining their smaller body size. However, Desai et al. (1984) found that such children had higher heart rates and lactic acid levels. They also found that a deficit of only one year in height and weight affected work performance at low levels of activity. This indicates that at more intensive levels of energy stress the adolescents would have to decrease the opportunity for exploration, discovery, and learning along with the effect on their physical growth and development. Thus, adolescent children adjusted to lower energy intake by first reducing weight gain; later, they reduced activity levels if malnutrition became more severe.

To what extent is any of this acceptable? A key finding is that parental management skills have a significant impact on children's nutritional status. Zeitlin, Mansour, and Bajrai (1987) have found in a review of past studies that mother-child interaction, their individual temperaments, and the social support network all have important implications for the child's nutritional outcome. Positive mother-child interaction would include the mother's meeting the child's needs, close physical holding and caressing, attention to socializing and safety instructions, absence of harsh punishments and controls, and creating a stimulating environment for the child. In addition, the social environment appears to favor efficient conversion of given nutrients into outcomes if the child's home includes a husband or male partner who is providing continuous support.

Later work shows that, even among moderately to severely undernourished children, as judged by weight-for-age, those with "normal developmental quotients" were much likelier to have "expressive" mothers than children with quotients below normal (Alvarez and Perez 1989). Thus "consistent differences in the competence of the mothers to provide child care might be present prior to the onset of undernutrition"[22] and (given the socioeconomic and demographic variables) strongly correlated both with avoidant and resistant child behavior and with undernutrition itself (Valenzuela 1974). Conversely, the much higher prevalence of sedatives, namely, opium and Phenargen, in diets of Iranian children whose mothers had a heavy workload seriously harmed their nutritional status despite higher family income (Rabiee and Geissler 1989, 226). In a coastal town in Pakistan, "women who are frequently sick are less competent in their child care activities," leading to worse child health and nutrition than in other households (Farhat Sultana 1989, 224). The traditional extended family in many developing countries may provide an important channel for consistent support in such circumstances. However, at least in most Indian villages (and especially among the poor, who are at greatest risk of energy stress), such extended family types are, and have long been, much rarer than is conventionally asserted (Shah 1979).

A comparison between better-nourished and worse-nourished children at school in rural Mexico revealed "that only one out of every 30 observations shows the [ill-nourished] child to be looking at the teacher attentively and that it is even rarer to find him obeying instructions . . . the poorly nourished child is passive . . . the supplemented child is more of a participant, is more interested, and is much more restless." In fact, most studies do show negative relationships between past and (especially) current nutritional status—on various measures[23]—and assorted indicators of school aptitude, learning, and attainment.

As to the causal processes involved, the situation is still uncertain. Chavez and Martinez (1982, 319) hypothesize that "malnutrition depresses activity, which in turn isolates the individual from . . . all sources of stimuli that are of vital importance to the functional development of the brain." Pollitt (1990), in a critical review, says of the current state of knowledge that ". . . the data gathered in the last 30 years are, at best, inconclusive; admittedly, not a single study can be cited that satisfies all the requirements of experimentation and at the same time provides a clear and distinct picture of the effects of early chronic undernutrition on mental development."

This has been partly remedied by a recent study—unique in its long duration (Pollitt et al. 1993)—of the long-term effects of food supple-

---

[22]Inquiry needs to be made as to whether it is unavoidable absence by mothers who need to work outside the home, not low maternal "competence," that reduces the child-care performance of some poor working women and hence their children's nutritional status. Such working mothers might be "negatively deviant" in child-care because they are forced by poverty and lack of productive assets to be "positively deviant" in leaving home to obtain income with which to feed their children. For examples of this, see Shekar, Habicht, and Latham (1989).

[23]One should, however, remember that current nutritional status, with respect to energy/protein, is likely to have been assessed simply by measuring current body size. Thus the distinctions between impact of past and current status, and between nutritional as opposed to other environmental causes, are unlikely to have been clearly demonstrated.

mentation during infancy. The study "in four villages of Guatemala . . . compared . . . the . . . effects of [a daily] Atole supplement [11.5 grams of protein; 163 kilocalories] or a Fresco supplement [59 kilocalories] on performance on a battery of psychoeducational and information-processing tests. [Persons supplemented] pre-natally and [aged 0-2 years were] contrasted with [those supplemented] only after 24 months." The effects of the feeding programs, carried out in 1969-77, were followed up (1) throughout the period and (2) in 1987 for adolescents and young adults up to age 24 (Pollitt et al. 1993: v, 26). The impact of age, gender, socioeconomic status, schooling variables (age of entry, leaving grade, attendance), and some "interaction variables" were separated from the impact of Atole vis-à-vis Fresco, that is, of extra food supplementation.

This study has its problems from the standpoint of evaluating responses, or adaptations, to dietary energy stress. This is not clearly the same as responses to "Atole instead of Fresco." First, the effects of Atole's extra dietary energy, protein, and micronutrients (as compared with Fresco) are not separable. Second, the level of home food intake—and therefore the effects, if any, on it of receiving Atole rather than Fresco—is unknown. In particular, "Fresco villages" even before 1969 inevitably differed in important ways—perhaps affecting food or health behavior or its changes in 1969-87—from "Atole villages." And relevant behavior of children or parents may have been affected by the fact that they, and the researchers, knew who received which supplement. However, Pollitt et al. (for example, pp. 74-75) honestly explore these problems, and their findings are telling for an understanding of cognitive adaptation to energy stress:

1. At most ages, regular childhood intake of Atole was associated with significant, persistent, but small gains in later mental performance. "The maximum accounted for by the Atole treatment was 5 percent (on the vocabulary tests) . . . [and] only about 1 percent of the variance [of] numeracy."

2. Atole was associated with a smaller proportion of variance (1-2 percent) in performance on information-processing tasks than on psychoeducational tasks (1-4 percent).

3. More performance variables are affected, at more age levels, and somewhat more substantially, for those whose mothers received Atole during pregnancy (and who received it in the first two years of life) than for those who received it only at ages 2-6.

4. The later the grade at which children left school, the larger was the effect of Atole on performance; indeed, on a separate sample of unschooled subjects (excluded from the main sample), "no effects of Atole were observed."

5. However, the lower the child's socioeconomic status, the larger was the effect of Atole.

Pollitt et al. argue that these effects are likely to result from behavioral modification linked to changes in nutritional status rather than from any direct, structural, or other functional changes in the brain or central nervous system resulting from improved diet. In their model, early nutrition directly influences physical size, motor development, and physical activity, all of which are crucial, not only to the development of exploratory and self-stimulating behavior but to the levels of interactive response with other individuals—especially with adult caregivers.

Suppose that the Atole-Fresco results can be applied to comparisons between subjects who are identical except in their exposure to dietary energy stress at various periods of life. If so, these results suggest that cognitive and behavioral "adaptation to stress" is in line with adaptation in characteristics such as height and in functional capacities such as physical performance and resistance to degenerative disease (Chapter 4). It seems that the prenatal period, together with the first two years of life, presents a "window of opportunity" for the growing child, in which the potential for future functional development is largely determined, but during which it is to some extent malleable and able to adapt to insult, at least if appropriately assisted. It is usually possible, in some degree, to recover from environmental insults—nutrient shortages, infectious diseases, or psychosocial deprivation—during later life; but as the "window" closes, it rapidly becomes difficult, if not impossible, to improve on the limits to the potential for development that were set earlier, whether these are for maximum stature or for cognitive achievement at maturity.

Pollitt et al. infer, from the strong interaction of food supplements with school grade levels, that removing the source of energy stress—by supplementary feeding for example—while necessary to improve potential, is, in contexts like Guatemala's, almost certainly insufficient to realize potential. "The school system, for example, is terribly inefficient and does not respond to the basic educational needs of the population. Less than half of the children enrolled in the first grade finish primary school, and many remain functionally illiterate. It is highly unlikely that the provision of food will prevent or remedy the consequences of not receiving an adequate formal education in a changing society." Even if partly biological, mechanisms of adaptation (including those triggered by supplementary feeding) may need to be "potentiated" by behavioral mechanisms—of schooling or parental care for example—if they are to improve outcomes, whether of bodily or mental performance.

If this interpretation of the research findings is correct, can it be concluded that learning behavior can always be acceptably adapted to cope with all but the most severe levels of energy stress? Probably not, because many parents lack the knowledge or resources to do what is necessary, not only to reverse the effects of the stress itself but also to dissociate them from linked, intellectually harmful features of the home environment. There can be distressing conflicts between family and child adaptation under stress. The Quechua Indians, at such times, rely *more* heavily on child labor for tasks involving mainly body translation; children's lightness, even more than small adults', increases the efficiency of conversion of food into tasks done (Thomas, cited in Smith 1979, 65).

Yet the balance of evidence is that extra calories alone, in infancy or at school, will not significantly improve the school aptitude, learning, or outcomes for mildly to moderately undernourished children. This appears to indicate that such children can tolerate strain from moderate calorie deprivation (on its own) without lasting intellectual damage. The role of "positive deviance" in home child care—shown in a Bangladesh study to relate to mother's education (holding wealth constant) via cleaner, more frequent child-feeding patterns (Guldan et al. 1989, 462)—is clearly important in facilitating such adaptive possibilities.

Food Acquisition and Composition

Changes in these behaviors, in order to avoid energy stress, often succeed to some extent but incur costs of other sorts. The most plausible options are to compress nonfood outlay (or non-food-acquiring activity) so as to obtain more food; to raise the proportion of cheap calories in food obtained; to draw on "food capital," notably livestock; to accept foods with high preservation or cooking costs or times, or with other unpleasant characteristics; or to enable family members to acquire more food by displacing household servants and doing the work themselves.

Those at most risk of energy stress, the poorest 15-25 percent of households in rural areas of low-income countries, typically devote some 80 percent of outlay (including self-consumed products) to food (Lipton 1983a). This "food share" is not readily increased when energy stress intensifies. If, as often happens, higher food prices are among the sources of such intensification, probably inducing some compression of the nonfood share, then the scope for further compression is usually very small. Less-poor people, however, do have this option.

What about sacrificing food diversity to obtain cheaper calories? Even the very poor sometimes have this option under stress (Shah 1983). More specific food composition choices involve turning, in hungry seasons, to larger amounts of foods that store well (even in drought) in the wild. These may be staples or more occasional foods; for example, mongongo nuts and melons for the !Kung (Lee 1973) and nuts and other foods for the Mbuti of eastern Zaire (Hart and Hart 1986). Other cases, for example among the Quechua Indians (Thomas, cited in Smith 1979, 65), involve trading protein foods, under stress, to acquire cheaper calories. In some cases in Papua New Guinea, such switches to cheap, low-protein foods appear to be associated with three bodily responses: the first within the lumen of the alimentary canal; the second involving mineral salts that increase the efficiency of protein turnover; and the third involving metabolic adjustments to low dietary intake of protein (Robson and Wadsworth 1977).

The extent and seasonality of infection critically determine whether such calorie-cheapening but protein-reducing changes, in avoiding energy stress, incur other severe costs. Where there are few seasonal infections the cost is less, as for the Ferlo in Senegal (Benefice, Chevassus-Agnes, and Barral 1984). Peak energy expenditure, however, coincides with malaria in Rosetta's (1986) group of Senegalese. An unusual suggestion by Lepowsky (1985) is that in Papua New Guinea, childhood food taboos on consumption of animal protein below weaning age may reduce the severity of malarial attacks among children aged about 6-36 months.[24] Murray et al. (1978) suggest a similar linkage between high-

---

[24]Such taboos may be a behavioral response to the need to keep energy sources cheap under stress.

protein diet and cerebral malaria in a nomad population in Niger consuming large quantities of milk. An outbreak of malaria followed refeeding after famine had restricted children to eating grain, not milk.

Often, accelerated livestock slaughter is the main way to avoid energy stress, for example, in the Mandara Mountains of northern Cameroon (Campbell and Trechter 1982) and among the Kenyan Masai (Campbell 1984). Whether such methods are sustainable depends on the division of net energy gains among and within households, on what happens if the source of stress is either unusually prolonged or unexpectedly repeated, and on how rapidly the livestock source is replenished (or replaced) after the stress period. At one extreme, if increased rates of cattle slaughter in hungry times are such as to irretrievably reduce herd size, this constitutes a "damage" response (see Chapter 2). At the other extreme, periodic, smaller increases of slaughter rates—typically due to rising grain-cattle price ratios and hence hungry times—not only "avoid" current energy stress, they reduce future risks by preventing overgrazing and permitting the bush to recover.

Cooking and preservation were central to Tswana selection of foods to avoid energy stress during drought (Grivetti 1978, esp. p. 120). Five factors were crucial: diversified food base, food preservation techniques, cooking methods, dietary practices, and food distribution methods. These mechanisms succeeded; despite the drought of 1965-72, in the period of Grivetti's research (1973-75) nutritional status was satisfactory.

Not all environments permit such apparently low-cost adaptation in food acquisition and composition. Although the ecology of the eastern Kalahari is semi-arid and subject to severe drought, it has great diversity of both vegetable and animal resources. In good times, the soils permit high yields of cultivated crops with only minor soil erosion on a flat landscape. The wild plants consumed by the inhabitants are remarkably high in calories, protein, fat, and vitamin C.

7

Who Is Stressed?
Who Adapts?

The questions of who is stressed and who adapts are addressed here only in regard to those issues relevant to research priorities on adaptation. Thus the large literature on socioeconomic and demographic causes of malnutrition is not reviewed in depth. The topic is divided in four possible ways to group people who might be subject to energy stress and then may or may not be able to adapt. First, energy stress and response may vary as between different socioeconomic groups such as landless, small farmer, and urban. Second, there is a small separate literature examining migration as a response to stress. Third, "the poor" may face different pressures or constraints in response to energy stress. Finally, many problems are special to particular physiological groups, especially infants and females. In the section on age and sex groups, the intrahousehold distribution of energy stresses and responses is briefly considered.

Socioeconomic Groups

Landed and Landless

Landless people are widely believed to be those at greatest risk of energy stress. They are indeed likeliest to face increased mortality rates in famines (Sen 1981; Drèze and Sen 1989). However, chronic risk of energy stress is clearly greater for the landless than for small farmers (with, say, 0.5-1.5 hectares to feed an average-size family) only where land and water conditions are relatively good. In semi-arid parts of India, command over food among the landless appears to be no worse than among persons owning or operating up to 5-7 acres. In parts of northern Nigeria, access to land may indicate absence of claims on more lucrative income sources and hence greater energy stress (Lipton 1985b).

Data on nutritional stress among landless families are not as plentiful as data on landed families. In Matlab thana, Bangladesh, landless mothers showed both lower average dietary energy intake and greater seasonal fluctuation than did mothers in landed families (Chen, Chowdhury, and Huffman 1980). For the landless, seasonal fluctuations in food prices (highest before harvest) often interact harmfully with seasonal fluctuations in participation rates and employment (Lipton 1983b). The latter were worse in their impact on the landless, as they are residual workers, likeliest to become unemployed in slack periods, while farm-family workers are retained.

Studies showing lower stress for the landed usually deal with rather fertile, often multicrop, lands (though often with very poor people). In semi-arid Indian areas with one crop per year, the operation of a little land—up to as much as 2-3 hectares—appears no likelier than landless-labor status to protect a household from earning so little income per person as to incur chronic nutrition stress (Visaria, cited in Lipton 1983b, 1985b). In similar areas, the International Crops Research Institute for the Semi-Arid Tropics (ICRISAT) has shown that seasonal variations in work and food—major sources of acute nutrition stress—are actually worse for farmers than for equally poor landless laborers (Walker 1984). Year-to-year acute variation, due to drought, had a similar pattern of incidence in semi-arid areas of rural Gujarat (Sambrani and Pichcholiya 1975). In general, however, land offers some protection against energy stress; if owned, it can at least be mortgaged.

More recent studies by IFPRI in the Philippines have shown that households that maintained access to land following the introduction of cash crops gained income and increased access to food (Bouis and Haddad 1988). However, for each household that gained, there was a tenant household that lost its access to land, and consequently lost reliable income, because the associated shift in the crop mix (from maize to sugar) neither increased nor stabilized the demand for labor. These households were especially exposed to energy stress because they would also have to expend additional energy in job search and commuting to work.

Preagriculture, Subsistence, and Cash-Crop Agriculture

Several pieces of research have looked at the transition from nomadic, tribal, or subsistence life-styles to settled or cash-crop economies, suggesting that the change has been for the worse. Gross and Underwood (1971) studied the impact on rural households in Brazil of the cash-cropping introduction. They found that cash cropping had been beneficial to landowners and entrepreneurs, as indicated by increased weight-for-height among their children. However, cash cropping had led to energy stress among farm laborers who had become landless. Farm labor required substantial extra energy expenditure by these laborers, which could be met only by allocating energy intake away from nonproductive dependents in the household, especially the children. Unfortunately, this study included no systematic analysis of energy stress conditions before cash cropping.

The effects on tribals apart, IFPRI's five-country study (von Braun and Kennedy 1986) and the Institute of Development Studies (IDS) review (Maxwell 1988) both show that the income and nutrition effects of the shift to cash cropping, even on the very poor, are usually favorable. Income gains outweigh higher transaction costs and risks of food consumption. However, at least in the short term, the reductions in energy stress for preschoolers are modest.

The literature on hunter-gatherers and archers suggests that they are not often under energy stress (on the Mbuti Pygmies, see Abruzzi 1979). In two studies, despite low calorie intake among a group of tribals

(Chitre, Deshpande, and Nimbalkar 1983; Pingale 1975), anthropological and clinical surveys indicated negligible nutritional deficiencies. Thus the considerable literature that interprets the subsistence strategies of these groups through the different amounts of energy consumed relative to the energy costs of foraging may not be relevant here.

A tiny but much-studied population, the hunter-gatherers (for example, in the Kalahari) do face nutritional stress and employ a set of strategies to adapt (Lee 1973; Bentley 1985). Such populations form a tiny part, well below 1 percent, of poor people in developing countries. A careful review of acculturation and settlement studies in Papua New Guinea (Dennett and Connell 1988) showed that prior to settlement the communities had often failed to adapt to nutrition stress, so that numbers declined—or adapted at plainly unacceptable cost in disease and child mortality—and also that gradual acculturation eased the constraints and was usually adapted to successfully, and welcomed by the adaptors.

Changes from tribal to settled life-styles are likely to compel nutritional change, often in respect of body composition (see "Changes in Body Composition" in Chapter 5). Among the Samburu in Kenya, a redistribution of body fat accompanied the transition from tribal to nontribal state. The nontribal members were engaged in a wider variety of duties; this more diversified activity may have led to the redeployment of the deposits of muscle and body fat (Day, Bailey, and Robinson 1979). The likely mechanism for such changes is that greater diversity of production or wage-earning opportunities results in smaller fluctuations in energy balance, even though average annual energy needs are increased—as seen, for example, in Burmese (as compared with West African) peasants (Dugdale and Payne 1987).

As for pastoralists, the Kenyan Turkana were studied by Galvin (1985) and found to have an extremely low energy intake level of 1,326 kilocalories per person per day. They buffered the apparent energy stress by a low level of energy expenditure. Eighty-one percent of the day is spent in "leisure activities." In addition, seasonal variations in energy intake were adapted to by some mixture of metabolic adaptation, body weight reduction, and fat loss. Not unexpectedly, for pastoralists as for tribals, in normal years the presence of spare land eases the task of adapting to energy stress. If population growth induces integration toward settled societies, the results are complex.

In an area of energy stress upon both farmers and pastoralists (Kajaido District of Kenya in 1972-76), it was difficult to sort out who was damaged by the resulting strain and who was adapting. Both types had strategies related to storage (of livestock and crops); stored products were exchanged, but there was little linkage at the ecological level, for example through complementary uses of land. "The effectiveness of [adaptive] strategies was related not only to the intensity of the drought, but also to their viability within a changing broader social, economic, and political environment" (Campbell 1984, 58). The constant movement of the Masai between herding and settled farming blurred any clear distinctions. In other words, it is the extent of (and constraints on) flexibility and complementarity between settled agriculture and its predecessor activities, probably more than the relative success and adaptability of each, that determines the relative and joint acceptability of farmers' and "pre-farmers'" adaptations to energy stress.

Urbanization and Community Change

Urban-rural differences in stress and adaptation are reviewed by Basta (1977). Clark (1980) showed rural Tongan children to be superior in terms of anthropometry to urban children, but this is very unusual. A review of the 12 national nutrition surveys carried out by the U.S. Agency for International Development (USAID) between 1975 and 1981 (Longhurst 1982) showed that rates of rural child malnutrition were on average twice the urban rates.

Traditional settled rural societies, such as the Mamainde of Brazil, sometimes have an exchange system that socially binds the village together in a common process of sharing (Aspelin 1979). The main mechanism of protection for the Tingalatar community in Nepal against the famine in 1971 was the interdependent Brahmin-Bhujel relationship. Famine was anticipated after repeated rain failure, and well-structured plans were formed at household and community levels. Wealthy farmers agreed not to sell grain outside the locality, and poorer households exchanged their daily products for cheaper, more filling carbohydrate sources such as millet (Prindle 1979). This sort of social contract is comparable with family-size adjustment under stress through temporary translation of individual members but should not be assumed to be general, especially where the rich no longer depend on labor from the poor because labor is less scarce or conditions less uncertain.

In analyzing who is stressed and who adapts, it may help to look at the Gemeinschaft-Gesellschaft distinction (Tonnies 1937). Throughout the world, there is a shift from the above traditional paternalistic insurance systems to modern social insurance systems. However, there is a period after the decline of the traditional insurance and prior to the introduction of the new system. In a society adopting modern technologies in farming, especially if they are labor-saving while the population and labor force are growing, the supply of traditional forms of insurance declines and demand for them goes up. Trust in new insurance systems does not form immediately; yet the rise in policing costs of old common property resources reduces their insurance role (Lipton 1985a). In this transitional period, there is increased risk of stress. Due to a rapidly changing social environment, biological and behavioral adaptations may also be slower to respond to stress, leading to increased chances of failure to adapt, at least acceptably.

Migrants

Migration is sometimes an adaptive response to nutritional stress. However, long-term migrants are usually better off nutritionally than the people with whom they settled, and seldom show signs of nutritional stress (Riley 1979, for Peru; Hull 1979; Schnetz, Egoramaiphol, and Leitzmann 1984, for Thailand; Black and Sanjur 1980, for Puerto Rico; Kashiwazaki 1983, for Bolivia).

The study of Desai et al. (1984) on migrant adolescent boys in Brazil did show some mild malnutrition. Also, de Almeida and Thomas (1989) find that Cape Verdean migrants to Lisbon undergo dietary changes that are "already contributing to . . . obesity and [the] risk of diabetes, cardiovascular disease and bowel disorders" in adults—but offsetting gains to infant growth and survival are not discussed. Of course, short-term seasonal migrants, homeless wanderers, and refugees are quite special groups, at very high risk of stress.

Income Groups

Does poverty expose its victims to particular types or levels of energy stress, of resulting strain, of consequent damage, or of responses (whether or not adaptive or acceptable)? For various reasons, poverty is more conveniently measured by outlay than by income (Glewwe and van der Gaag 1988). Also, because households with low outlay may not be poor if they also have few members (or few adult consumers), it is essential to assess a household's poverty, not by its total outlay (Datta and Meerman 1980) but by its outlay per person—or better, if available, by household outlay per adult-equivalent consumer, or HOPAEC. Does this reveal much about household energy stress and adaptation?

There are two extreme ways to interpret that question to which clear answers exist. First, is there a strong positive relationship (high response elasticity and high correlation coefficient)—over the whole range of HOPAEC from the severest destitution up to a comfortable level of living—between a lower level of HOPAEC and probability of shortfall, among that household membership, either below (say) WHO/FAO/UNU-indicated intakes relative to requirements or below (say) NCHS median height-for-age in children or weight-for-height in adults? Increasingly clearly, the answer is no. Such relationships are strong only below a low threshold level of HOPAEC, different in different sorts of households and communities. As HOPAEC rises above that level, preferences for dietary variety and other attributes loom very large, relative to preferences for extra calories, unless the extra HOPAEC is being achieved through extra effort rather than higher returns per unit of effort (Bouis and Haddad 1988; Behrman and Deolalikar 1988).

Second, is there a level of HOPAEC such that, below it but not otherwise, there is a substantial risk that energy intakes are so seriously below requirements as to lead to severe anthropometric shortfalls—and hence to major increases in risk of reduced mental or working capacity, of illness, or even, among preschoolers, of death? Increasingly clearly, the answer is yes.

In their study of Nicaragua, Behrman and Wolfe (1984) found an extremely weak positive relationship between nutritional intake and HOPAEC. Their income elasticities of demand for energy were very small (though inversely related to HOPAEC). Also, mother's education was found to have a highly significant positive relationship with nutritional demand. In other words, low mother's education could be a better indicator of energy stress than low HOPAEC. However, this appears to be likely only at "Latin American" income levels, where the rather low food-outlay ratios among poverty groups (for example, 40 percent at the official poverty line in Brazil, as against over 70 percent in India) suggest that, except among those well below the poverty line, not many people are hungry for want of income.[25]

In much poorer areas, Lipton (1983a) reported several microstudies and sample surveys in which measured income elasticities or expenditure elasticities of demand for food among "ultrapoor households"—typically those spending around 80 percent of outlay on food, yet failing to meet even 80 percent of FAO/WHO (1973) energy intake recommendations—were not significantly below unity. Such households typically reduced neither the proportion of outlay devoted to food nor the staples-food ratio as total household income and outlay rose, as long as HOPAEC remained below a critical level—behavior violating the Engel and Bennett laws, respectively.[26] While this does not prove that demand for energy is highly responsive to increasing HOPAEC even at these very low levels, such behavior strongly suggests that perceived energy stresses are important in, and confined to, these very poor groups (Edirisinghe and Poleman 1983).

Violation of Engel's Law at extremely low levels of HOPAEC is confirmed in Edirisinghe and Poleman 1983 and in Bhanoji Rao 1981. They found that, among the poorest 15-25 percent of households surveyed, rising HOPAEC does not appear to induce a falling proportion of outlay on food in general, or even on starchy staples. Strauss and Thomas (1990) have examined several data sets to disprove the view that this "violation" of Engel's Law is an artifact produced by a few outrider observations.

Above the threshold, as HOPAEC rises further, households diversify their purchases away from basic food staples. This suggests that there is no longer perceived energy stress. However, while this clearly differentiates the ultrapoor (or food-poor) from others, the relationship of HOPAEC to energy acquisition per adult-equivalent consumer over the whole income range is weaker. In rural areas of five less-developed countries, recent IFPRI work (von Braun and Kennedy 1986) shows weak (though positive) links between HOPAEC and short-run energy balance, anthropometry, or health outcomes in preschoolers. Except at very low levels of HOPAEC, it appears to be "loosely meshed" rather than "tightly wedded" to dietary energy intake and to nutritional status, at least in the short term (Behrman 1988a). This does not prove that people at higher HOPAEC—above the poorest quintile or so in India or Africa—correctly perceive themselves to be nutritionally adapted and in

---

[25]It might be mentioned that women's schooling and HOPAEC are likely to be positively related. However, if this produced strong collinearity between them as explanatory variables of energy intake, then their statistical significance (t-statistics) would be low, which is not the case in Behrman and Wolfe 1984. However, that could be explained by a nonlinear positive relationship between women's schooling and HOPAEC.

[26]Engel's Law states that, as HOPAEC rises, the proportion spent on food falls; Bennett's, that the proportion of food outlay devoted to starchy staples falls.

need of few extra calories when HOPAEC rises further.[27] However, the important exception to loose meshing—that energy intake does rise substantially, even above the threshold, when HOPAEC and labor input increase together—does suggest that the loose meshing rule may represent a correct perception among households above a community-specific HOPAEC threshold (Lipton 1989).

To the extent that low HOPAEC is passed from generation to generation, notably among "hereditary" outgroups in low-income countries (for example, *harijan* castes in India), various forms of adaptation may be associated with poverty itself. These permit survival and possibly, but not necessarily, full functioning. Laborers too undernourished to work are at evolutionary disadvantage, so that "food-economizing" genomes may be selected among the hereditarily poor. However, neither this nor behavioral adaptation by the poor is an unmixed advantage for them. "Families living under conditions of extreme poverty generally adapt to this condition, and are not entirely aware of the abnormality of their situation . . . . For them, the malnourished child is not the consequence of poverty . . . . They find explanatory factors inherent to the child and not the environment (the child is weak, or ill)" (Riumallo and Monckeberg 1983). Long-run adaptation, if it confers low expectations, can in such circumstances impede short-run recovery.

Age and Sex Groups

Although it is clear that nutritional stress somehow gets "allocated" within an affected family, there has been substantial debate over how this is accomplished. In particular, is hardship reflected in allocations of dietary energy that are, in some appropriate sense, proportional to requirements? Or does the intrahousehold distribution of access to food reflect repartitioning, that is, unequal distribution of either chronic or acute hardship between individual household members? In chronic stress, some limits can be placed on the degree of "maldistribution" likely to be common by the observation by Clarke and Haswell (1970) of the remarkable constancy of the grain equivalent of the minimum agricultural wage. They found ". . . throughout all times and places for which we have information, the rural labourer, however poor, will not do a day's work for less than three kilograms grain equivalent." Seckler (1980), confirming that this figure holds good for Indian laboring households of average size, observed that it is substantially above the level at which, assuming the wage-earner continued to meet his physiological needs, the lives of his dependents would be seriously threatened. Seckler concluded that the almost universal minimum of 3 kilograms makes sense only on the basis of one crucially important assumption, which he found "entrancing," that wage-earners love their

---

[27]Perceptions may be incorrect partly because a head of household, when income rises, makes judgments about the unmet energy requirements of other household members, including inarticulate infants.

dependents to the extent that they will "irrationally" share their scarce food supplies in proportion to their needs rather than treating them as residual claimants.

While this might be true for the average, there may of course be exceptions. It has often been claimed that, particularly during periods of stress, women suffer more than men and children more than adults. Recent literature has shown the situation to be less clear-cut.

First, even if there were relatively more attention to maintaining nutrition for some age or sex groups, it might maximize the proportion of a total population that survives or avoids serious harm. This would be the case if such favored groups were at greater risk, as seems to be the case with boys in regard to mental damage from undernutrition (Lipton 1983a, 52). Overall survival prospects could also increase if energy stress were "kept away" from family members who had to engage in a risky search for uncertain wage work, and who could feed other household members (from wages) only if a job could be found and completed.

Second, discrimination against children or females in nutrition appears to be the exception, not the rule. A study in Guatemala reveals one reason the opposite is often asserted; indeed, "adult males are favoured in the distribution of kcals at regular mealtimes, [but] children . . . when total daily consumption is calculated . . . cultural rules . . . favouring males . . . seem to operate at formal meal events only. Feeding behaviour between meals . . . tends to compensate by favouring those not favoured" at mealtimes (Nieves and Engle 1989). Mothers and children adapt, by avoidance of the source of stress, to male dominance as a source of food shortages. Hence a comprehensive review of intra-family distribution of hunger in South Asia attributed malnutrition much more to lack of household entitlement than to maldistribution within the household (Harriss 1986, esp. p. 46).

Third, even in places where this is not normally true, it becomes true in extreme conditions. A recent careful study in Bangladesh (Abdullah and Wheeler 1985) showed significant seasonal differences in energy intake for adults and for young children aged 1-4 years. Seasonality, however, did not exacerbate these differences absolutely, that is, it reduced them relatively.

Overall, it is rare for children not to receive the share of household food that requirements would prescribe, or for young girls to receive a significantly lower share than young boys. Serious and widespread examples are reported only in parts of northern India and Bangladesh and are refuted for Africa and Latin America (Harriss 1986; Lipton 1983a; Svedberg 1989, esp. chap. 7; Schofield 1979). Where such discrimination does happen, as in Bangladesh, it almost has to be corrected when food supply is shortest, in times of special stress; indeed, young girls' share then increases (Abdullah and Wheeler 1985). The study concluded that intrahousehold allocation does follow the same pattern as expected requirements, except for the youngest children. Children of all ages were given more calories per kilogram of body weight than adults. There was no consistent difference in nutritional status (weight-for-age) between boys and girls. Therefore, in one of the (exceptional) countries where discrimination against girls in nutrition is clearly proven (Chen,

Huq, and D'Souza 1981)—though probably due to differential health care, not food intake—corrections are made in the worst seasons, both away from sex differentials and away from preferential food allocation for working males. However, the latter has been found in populations where such males faced job search in the stressed season, by Chen, Huq, and D'Souza (1981) in Bangladesh and by Behrman (1988b, 1988c), working with a South Indian data set.

Such seasonal corrections have also been shown for weanlings in Bangladesh (Brown et al. 1985). Discrimination against girls below 2 years of age was not apparent during the season of greatest nutritional stress; but the postharvest improvement in intakes was greater and began earlier among the older (18-30 months) boys. This appears to be due to the greater consumption of breast milk as well as rice. For both boys and girls, energy intake was approximately one-third greater during the postharvest period than during the preharvest period. Therefore, weanlings in Bangladesh were heavily affected by seasonal changes in food production and availability, but sex discrimination again declined during the severest stress.

In the two populations studied by Norgan, Ferro-Luzzi, and Durnin (1982), the energy intake of adult men (relative to apparent FAO/WHO/UNU requirements) was higher than that of women—a rather unusual finding (Schofield 1979, Lipton 1983a)—but this difference was reduced or reversed in the groups of older children.

In exceptional cases where protein-energy malnutrition is clearly more prevalent among females, for example in some poor rural communities in Mexico, undernourished males may have been absent from the samples because they were already dead; more undernourished females were found because they were more resistant. The female infant grows less with the same amount of protein, but this may have a positive aspect because the consumption of the same amount of milk for a smaller body would contribute to her survival. Males may convert protein "better," grow faster, and either survive and grow to higher anthropometric levels or die (de Chavez et al. 1974, who conclude that this hypothesis is not proven).

The hypothesis that women are better adapted to surviving seasonal stress has been supported not only by the cognition literature (see "Cognition" section in Chapter 5) but also by Rosetta's (1986) study in Senegal. Here the men, especially those over 55, showed a seasonal mobilization of muscle mass (that is, a reduction to "feed" the remaining tissues, indicated by changes in lower-arm circumference) during the rainy season, whereas the women resisted seasonal food stress more than men (regardless of their age and physiological status) without mobilizing muscle mass. Men less than 55 years of age lost 2.7 percent, and those over 55 years, 4.8 percent, of their body weight. The lower-arm circumference of women remained in equilibrium whatever the season, with the exception of one year of the three-year study.[28] The

---

[28]However, even in this year the absolute value of the decreases was lower than in the male groups.

reasons for this are not clear. One reason for the weight loss in men may be sex-related differences in work distribution, that is, that only the men increase energy expenditure during the stressed season; but this involves training effect and is hard to reconcile with reduced muscle mass.

Rosetta's (1986) study was carried out in periods of severe seasonal stress—virtually famine conditions. These may involve a "pecking order" in communities in terms of casting off family members. Families disintegrate with children being sent away to other families (or even sold) and the elderly left behind. Dirks (1980) confirms that during famine the very young and old are in greatest jeopardy; the health of both groups deteriorates rapidly. The 1939 famine in the Punjab brought considerable increases in death rates for those under 10 years and over 60 years, while the death rates of those aged 10-60 declined, probably because they were better able to move in search of food or work.

8

Conclusions and Proposals for Research

Conclusions

This review has considered two basic questions. First, what biological and behavioral mechanisms do individuals, households, and larger population groups use in adapting to the challenge of different sources, intensities, and durations of energy stress? Second, given that successful adaptation implies only that the chances of an individual's surviving to contribute to the inheritance of future generations are improved or maintained, what counterbalancing costs are incurred and who suffers most from these?

The particular combinations and timing of stresses and responses vary widely. Responses differ according to types of livelihood, family structures and stage of development, ecological settings, and cultural traditions. The origins and timing of the stress itself also affect the range of feasible and appropriate adjustments.

The rich diversity of these patterns of response makes for both the difficulty of the subject and its importance for policy. The strategies that families normally adopt to avoid, repartition or resist, or tolerate undernutrition have to be understood in order to find effective ways of helping them with the adoption. Indeed, an outsider's strategies may merely disrupt or displace their older coping mechanisms, especially if such strategies represent responses to long climatic cycles or even to the experience of regular drought (Morris 1974). Neither, without understanding such strategies, can policymakers allocate scarce nutritional and health resources in the public domain efficiently, for this requires the ability to estimate, at least roughly, the places, times, and circumstances in which the capacity to respond to stress without unacceptable damage to health or livelihood is likely to be exceeded.[29]

More effective policy choices for prevention, either through strengthening and extending existing traditional adaptive strategies or through better targeting of relief toward those for whom such strategies are not acceptable or whose options have run out, will require more

---

[29]If moderately to severely undernourished families respond to increased energy stress by redistributing food toward (potentially) employed family members, they may reduce the survival prospects of living children but increase the family's chance to pull through as a self-reproducing unit in the long run.

than just the recognition of diversity. The manifold adjustments that households make in the face of energy stress are not simply random. It should be possible to distinguish consistent patterns: hierarchies, distributions, and time sequences of changes that can be thought of as a variety of strategies of response.

It may be useful to spell out a little more fully one example of the consequences of the "adaptation-acceptability" approach taken here at individual and household levels. In the matter of intrahousehold distribution, the notion is rejected that the needs of individual family members are fairly met if, and only if, their expected intakes are proportional to the average, or expected, requirements for the age, sex, and activity level of the groups to which each member belongs. Such average requirements can indeed be estimated as recommended by successive WHO/FAO committees. Until recently, however, this has been done without reference to the specific context.[30] In particular, a household or set of households that allocates a particular age- or sex-group "more than its fair (average) share" of calories should be assumed, until the contrary is proven, to face either or both of two conditions: (1) an above-average requirement of energy in that group (for example, to do or seek work, to fight infection, to insure against the risk of these, or even to support an unusually high RMR), and (2) a more significant impact, for that group, of extra dietary energy on anthropometric status, as in the case of boys vis-à-vis girls in Guatemala (Martorell et al. 1980, 225).

Therefore, data on actual food consumption (or its changes) by age- and sex-groups within a household, expressed as a proportion of such groups' average expected requirements (or their changes), does not tell us much about equity or the lack of it between adults and children or between males and females. Unfairness or discrimination of food sharing could be determined only on the basis of concurrent measurements of both intakes and expenditures of energy. Some assessment of outcome should also be required in terms of the nutritional status of the household members and its impact on their contribution to household resources. Finally, as the evidence in this study underlines, it is necessary to know who—male or female, young or old—is likeliest to fail in adapting to various sources of energy stress. Very few studies provide this kind of data. As it happens, those that most closely approach the ideal seem to show that, in regard to regular and predictable seasonal stress, discrimination is if anything in favor of children, even in favor of girl children. Furthermore, if anything, men show greater seasonal changes in weight status than women. Women are likelier than men (in small samples with energy expenditures carefully measured) to show longish periods of apparent negative energy balance without weight loss (Edmundson and Edmundson 1989), confirming the Dunn team's conclusion (Dunn Nutrition Unit 1986; Nestlé Foundation 1987, 1988) that

---

[30]FAO/WHO/UNU (1985) moves a long way toward allowing for context, at least as regards activity levels, but leaves the reader hard-pressed to rank persons, communities, or areas in order of need at all, given the limited data usually available.

women—and not only (though very powerfully) in pregnancy and lactation—have more effective means of metabolic adjustment.

In response to severe and unpredictable stress, there is evidence of discrimination against the very young and the very old after prolonged famine. As a last resort, death risks to these groups are allowed by desperate households to increase so as to improve the prospects for reproductive and potentially self-sufficient household members and thus for the household as a whole. However, in traditional societies at least, this happens only after the scope for adjustment through sharing of food, fuel, time, and other resources within and between households has been exhausted. In other words, the sequence "avoidance-repartitioning-resistance" has been followed through to the point of tolerance of damage. At this point, however, survival of those most likely to succeed in rebuilding the household is perhaps seen as the first priority.

Where falls in income, rather than famines or seasonal patterns, are the source of stress there are again problems of incompleteness of data from which to draw inferences about what changes households choose and in response to what stresses. A 10 percent income fall that is linked to a big fall in energy expenditure as a result of a similar fall in employed work, for instance, provides a much smaller energy stress, and would be expected to induce much less fall in calorie intake, than a similar income fall with no remission in working intensity. Yet generally one is forced to try to draw conclusions about "responses to income-induced energy stress" from household cross-sections (more rarely time series) showing differences (or changes) in income or total expenditure and in household average consumption of energy and other nutrients without knowledge of concomitant changes in energy expenditure. Usually the evidence is of positive but unexpectedly small elasticities of energy intake in response to changes in income for, or differences in income across, households of given age-sex composition, even in rather poor communities. However, there are probably discontinuities—not merely nonlinearities—in such variations of behavior,[31] which mirror similar breakpoints in the otherwise smooth operation of Engel's and Bennett's laws of consumption.[32] Evidently, when a decline in income is a source of energy stress, the decision about whether to adjust energy acquisition down, or to do something else instead, involves complex shifts of behavior and redistributions of consumption, with substantial differences among families having similar levels of income, depending on such factors as different types of employment and access to health improvements.[33]

---

[31]See Strauss and Thomas 1990 for recent strong evidence from Brazil of income elasticities of demand for calories around 0.25-0.30 for people in the poorest decile of expenditure per person but much lower for others (and "at the mean"): see also Behrman 1990 and Bouis and Haddad 1990.

[32]On these, see Lipton 1983a, Bhanoji Rao 1981, and Edirisinghe and Poleman 1983.

[33]If child welfare is so constrained by bad health-sanitation-care environments that extra calories do little for it, then even very poor households may be forced to conclude that there is little gain from feeding more to children (or to their parasites and bacteria) when income rises.

Evidence of the nutritional outcome of such adjustments, that is, of changes in nutritional status, is also frustratingly limited in the large majority of cases to measurements on small children. What can justifiably be inferred from these measurements about the nature of intrafamily adjustments? The conclusion here is that current views on the nature of the causes of growth retardation in children do not support the use of child anthropometry as a proxy for household food (energy) availability. Only if health-sanitation environments, adult work energy requirements, genetics, and medical histories of two sets of households were both "normal," or otherwise both closely similar or well controlled for, could differences in child anthropometry be confidently attributed to differences between the two communities in household energy availability or in the success of adjustments to it.

Of course, an individual child who is smaller than expected for its age must have received or retained less energy (or complementary nutrients), relative to its requirements, than a "normal" healthy person. However, to suggest that such smallness measures the extent to which undernutrition was a cause of it is seriously misleading. The cause of poor growth may have been almost any combination or sequence over time of factors such as illness, infectious or otherwise; emotional stress; neglect; abuse; orphanhood; or even low birth weight or genetic factors. Restriction of food offered to the child might be a main or contributory cause of that poor growth, but it is by no means a necessary one. Thus the presence or the frequency of smallness for age among children should not be expected to bear any consistent relationship to the current or past level of food availability in the households to which those children belong.

Moreover, a pattern of reduced growth (especially in length or height), once established for whatever reason, becomes difficult to reverse after the first one or two years of life. Thus, even in those cases where food restriction is known to have been a major cause, removal or reduction of that stress may produce at most only a rather small recovery in expected size for age. Parents whose inherited wisdom suggests that this applies to their own children may rationally respond to increases in income by raising children's food intake much less than other parents would do, thus dragging down observed income elasticities of children's energy intakes for the sample as a whole but not necessarily for those households where a high responsiveness matters greatly for children's well-being.

This model of "rational adaptation" or "health-seeking behavior" (Alderman 1993) has two implications. First, taken together with the complexity of the intrahousehold adjustments already noted, it explains why such a small proportion of interhousehold variability in child anthropometric status is explained by differences in such sources of stress as household expenditure per head. Second, it means that, as part of an adaptive strategy for dealing with energy stress, it is necessary to distinguish short-run, more or less directly mediated responses—such as body weight loss consequent upon and compensating directly for negative energy balance—from longer-run, lifetime processes in which general environmental stress in very early life leads to a sustained reduction in body size. These can be regarded as anticipatory components of lifetime energy-saving strategies for dealing with an environment in which the risk of energy stresses of various kinds is likely to be high, and in which a sharp fall in food intake (leading to energy stress) is a particularly likely source (see "Smallness as a Direct Contribution to Energy-Saving" in Chapter 5).

Of all the biological responses made by individuals, those related to changes of body size are probably the most significant, both in terms of the amount of energy saved through size/weight reduction and in regard to the relatively small costs incurred. Size changes are adaptive: people bad at making such changes at low cost under energy stress (for example, very lean people) are at relatively greater risk. The evidence also suggests that changes large enough to contribute very significant savings of energy, either in face of short-term stress or as part of a lifetime strategy, often result in rather small losses of functional capacity. In particular this seems likely to be the case for work capacity, especially if weight reduction is part of an integrated response that includes behavioral changes resulting in increased efficiency of task accomplishment through changes of timing or intensity of work or both. Such changes probably include selection of tasks (involving, for example, much body translation and little lifting of weights) suitable to small people or to people especially exposed to the risk of weight loss.

Social policy as well as research and training policy has its part to play in ensuring that earning capacity and employment in these "small people's tasks" are advanced in the development process. Labor intensity is usually essential if a production system is to provide adequate food entitlements on average to the very poor; but great caution is desirable in order to avoid forms of "effort intensity" that favor large and muscular people if, as appears to be necessary, a part of development strategy is to sustain adaptive capacities.

Compared with size changes, other biological components of response, such as altered body composition, changes in thermogenesis, and what has been termed "metabolic adaptation," result in relatively smaller energy savings when considered separately. Also, there is more uncertainty (than for modest changes in body size) as to whether in any given set of circumstances any of these involves bearable (much less acceptable) costs. Insofar as all of them are likely to take place together as part of an integrated response, their contribution may be a small but significant addition to the effect of size changes operating alone.

Returning to the issue of "big is better" versus "small is beautiful," no good reason to take either side has been found. None of the evidence reviewed here suggests a general advantage of bigness per se. For example, the argument that irreversible lifetime reductions in height might "close off" future options for which tallness might have some (unforeseen) advantage is not persuasive. And smallness might, for other options, have unforeseen relative advantages. It is apparent, however, that where small size is the outcome of environmental stresses at any period of life, those adverse processes that result in smallness are not acceptable, even if the people who survive them are not further disadvantaged by reason of their size. Thus this study supports the view that smallness is both adaptive and acceptable but that it is nevertheless important, often urgent, to interrupt the process of becoming small. Scar tissue may be an adaptive and acceptable response to burning; burning itself is neither adaptive nor acceptable.

A caution should be added, however. Whether or not bigness has advantages, adult body size will be increased, not only by economic development (which causes parents to spend more on children's food and health), but also by government activities to promote child growth. If such activities succeed, they will greatly increase the future food needs of the adult population. It is irresponsible to ignore these outcomes or to discount them on the grounds that bigger people will somehow be more productive of food (or items exchangeable for it) and will have more access to the food when needed. Unless there is a clear and secure basis for sustainably larger and widely available future food supplies, and for the adults to earn access to them via increased activity to produce food or food-exchangeables, the larger adults will tend to become either wasted (tall but hungry) or idle (poor but fat). Both outcomes may be worse than a "small but not very unhealthy" adulthood.

This study has established a wide range of biological responses to several forms of energy stress. The authors hope to use Indian data, and new studies based on them, to establish how far these differences mean that some households "do better" than others, that is, that some sorts of private or social behavior give better chances for the biology of response to stress to be in the first place adaptive and, in addition, acceptable. Inquiries to that end, however, have raised a further issue that complicates this plan of work.

Behavioral responses—especially via the quantity, intensity, duration, type, and ergonomics of work done—are, because they are in general more flexible and rapidly available, likely to be more important immediate adjustments to energy stress than are biological responses, even including the most important of these (reduced body size or growth). Yet behavioral responses interact with biological responses in complex ways. For example, if a man responds to food shortage by working less, his potential for biological adjustments (from weight loss to BMR reduction) is hardly tested. On the other hand, some behavioral responses render particular adjustments more likely or amplify or even cause them; when hungry people can adapt by reducing very vigorous activity, they save energy not only directly but also (probably) by reducing RMR per kilogram and the thermic effect of feeding. Another interaction is that behavioral responses— who in a household works less during a period of energy stress?—can repartition biological response: who else in the household loses weight? Such interactions, together with evidence on the effects of alternative biological responses and judgments on acceptability, greatly affect policy choices. It should be assumed that people, especially hungry people, respond rationally to policy changes affecting food.

Proposals for Further Research

Policy Processes and Nutrition Research

Although an arcane discussion about the general problem of defining objectives, social relevance, and priorities for research is avoided here, something needs to be said about the categories into which it might be useful to divide this potentially extensive range of topics.

There is a general presumption that relevance to national policies should be an important criterion for identifying research priorities. However, the nature of the policy process itself is usually left undefined and is treated as exogenous to the research process and its outputs. For example, the United Nations' Sub-Committee on Nutrition (of the Administrative Committee on Coordination) convened an ad hoc working group in 1986 to consider the possibility of devising a systematic schema for identifying research areas related to "defining nutritional problems, solving them, and implementing the solutions." However, the issues considered were essentially related to the best uses of science within policy. There was no discussion of the possible impacts of research on the policy process itself.

The apparent research priorities on adaptation to dietary energy stress have emerged in a somewhat piecemeal fashion throughout this review. Before they are pulled together, three guidelines will be suggested for choosing types of research that will help to improve the policy process by rendering it more responsive to the priorities of people at nutritional risk.

1. A wide range of policies is likely to affect whether a group of people is able to adapt to the types of energy stress that it experiences and to do so in ways acceptable both to the group at risk and to society as a whole. Moreover, the types of feasible policy as well as the sources of stress and the adaptive processes all differ over time and space. Therefore, even leaving aside the issue of possible differences in moral preferences among persons and groups, the acceptability (or otherwise) of the outcomes will depend heavily on the particular context. This applies not only to programs that are designed to affect specific nutritional inputs but also to those that are in the first place aimed at nonnutritional objectives but may nonetheless have nutritional outcomes. The scope for establishing general rules for nutrition policy in all cases, as distinct from rules for selecting a type of nutrition strategy suitable to particular types of circumstances, is small. Therefore, the reduction of unacceptable outcomes of energy stress implies current, location-specific research, iterating with continuous assessment, adjustment, and monitoring of change.

2. The at-risk group's current ethical values and capacity to manage social adjustments are part of the context. Each population group, and its political system, needs research to enable it to establish and prioritize its concerns about the levels of deprivation—and means of adaptation—that it deems unacceptable in the light of the social and economic costs implied by their reduction. Yet current agenda-setting for research, into adaptation to dietary energy stress for example, generally begins with

advocacy (often by international groups) of externally perceived impera-
tives and priorities assessed on the basis of "global" indicators and
targets. What is needed is to shift the goals of policy research away from
identifying researchable (that is, technically soluble) "problems" for all
circumstances toward categorizing types of conditions where particular
sorts of problems arise and where particular types of solution are
appropriate; away from implementing "solutions" on the basis of cen-
trally determined goals toward using the procedures of civil society for
goal-setting; and away from top-down models that yield "optimizing"
outcomes toward open, pluralist ways to help people to influence and
manage the *processes* affecting their own nutrition, health, and capabilities. This refers not only to the processes involved in adaptation, but also
to the processes by which ethical standards are evolved, discussed, and
translated into political compromises and priorities for allocating scarce
resources.

The State of Oregon wants to help its own voters—taking note of,
but not subordinate to, the judgments of medical scientists—to decide
on the priorities for publicly supported health care. In poor countries,
where resources are scarcer and where there are more serious unmet
needs (including nutritional inadequacies), a similarly democratic process of prioritizing public responses to energy stress is even more
strongly indicated. Adaptation research should seek to inform that
process.

3. Useful research, however basic at first, should ultimately improve
the understanding of the capacities that some, but not all, people or
groups possess for adjusting successfully, and even acceptably, to energy
stress. One example is the study of "positive deviance" as a factor in
child survival.

Aims of Research

Against this background, the overall aims of research become easier to
define. First, more information is needed about what types of individuals, households, and communities are prone to various sources of energy
stress. To what extent does the sustainability of their livelihoods depend
upon their ability to make effective adjustments in response to the
resulting stresses? Second, research should help to distinguish the different types and scope of responses they make. What is the relative strategic importance of these along the sequence of avoidance, repartitioning,
resistance, or tolerance? Third, research should help to reveal the
mechanisms and processes involved. What are the limits beyond which
further adjustment ceases to be adaptive, that is, ceases to maintain
biological fitness?

Research on adaptation to energy stress, then, should improve the
sorts of understanding that can help at-risk groups not only to make
better personal choices but also to apply their own (evolving) preferences to influence and improve policies that have nutritional outcomes.
In that perspective, an underlying concern derives from the attempt in
this report to clarify disputes about the existence and extent of adaptive
processes. As defined here, adaptation must, in the nature of things,

exist—and in a wide variety of forms. Research may well show that some of these forms, or the strategies through which they are deployed, are relatively minor in scope.

More seriously for this perspective on research as a means toward informed participation, it may turn out that some adaptations cause, or are strongly associated with, quite severe costs. (This is known to be the case for severe growth retardation in children, for example.) However, the criteria by which such responses or strategies are judged on balance to contribute to rather than detract from biological fitness, that is, to be adaptive, lie firmly within the realm of evolution through natural selection. A particular outcome might be adaptive, yet could be shown by research to be unacceptable given existing social values, and avoidable given available resources. Equally, some outcomes currently regarded as acceptable might prove to imply hidden costs that render them nonadaptive and, if those newly perceived costs are to individual health or survival prospects, unacceptable as well.

Ideology inevitably influences research priorities. Also, almost every aspect of adaptation to dietary energy stress is characterized by some lack of knowledge. Nevertheless, an attempt has been made in this study to prioritize research areas that appear to offer relatively high prospects of success per research dollar and of empowerment of hungry people to take (and to press for) better decisions per "unit of success."

A few examples of such research topics are given below under four categories.

- *People, Risks, and Sources*

  To establish methods for identifying groups—by age, sex, infection history, and perhaps environmental or ethnic background—that are, either on average or for the lower quartiles by income or nutritional status, particularly badly able to adapt at low cost to dietary energy stress.

  To establish methods for distinguishing which of the possible different sources of stress is directly responsible for (as distinct from associated with) the (1) strain or damage, or (2) high-cost adaptive responses. In particular, when is infectious disease, as distinct from household food availability, the source of stress responsible for minimally damaging reductions in child growth, more seriously damaging reductions, or increasing mortality?

  To determine the contributions of genetic and environmental factors to the observed differences between population groups in the level of mortality risk associated with the same degree of deficit below international child growth standards and below adult height and BMI norms.

- *Types and Strategies of Adaptation*

  To examine whether birth cycles and a tendency to increase rest in pregnancy, as adaptations to dietary energy stress or the risk of it, are behavioral or biological (the policy implications of such research could extend well beyond nutrition education).

To assess the scope of existing, and perhaps additional, responses of working methods to various forms and degrees of dietary energy stress among different sorts of affected workers; the costs in health, comfort, output, or earnings of such responses; and how to reduce such costs where they are significant.

To examine whether the provisional finding that there is a small but clear effect on BMR of over- or underfeeding carries through to larger trials and, most especially, whether the same effect occurs in children.

- *Mechanisms, Processes, and Limits*

  To examine the role of energy-saving behavioral adaptation at the household level, in particular the alteration of the household cycle in order to improve food security when the threat of drought or famine overlaps with a household-specific high risk, such as a demographic composition in which there are several small children and only one working adult.

  To test the scope of the findings now suggesting that metabolic adaptation during lactation is "proportionate to need," that is, that ethnic backgrounds, and environments, likely to be energy-stressed adapt more than others. (At a later stage, analogous hypotheses could be tested for other groups; the initial research is now especially promising for lactating women.)

  To examine the effects of current and previous anthropometric status on adult risks of illness and infection (occurrence, duration, and attendant risks).

  To replace or to complement existing cut-off points for anthropometric classifications, which are based on normative distributions, with ones based on context-specific risk thresholds.

- *Acceptability*

  To explore carefully the existence and extent of adverse side effects of adaptations such as increased metabolic efficiency under energy stress.

  To examine whether there are decisions that individuals, households, communities, or policymakers at local and national levels can take that will increase capacity to adapt metabolism or thermogenesis to energy stress, or that will lower the costs of such adaptation, if any.

Bibliography

Abdullah, M., and E. Wheeler. 1985. Seasonal variations and the intra-household distribution of food in a Bangladeshi village. *American Journal of Clinical Nutrition* 41: 1305-1313.

Abruzzi, W. 1979. Population pressure and subsistence strategies among the Mbuti Pygmies. *Human Ecology* 7 (2): 183-189.

Alderman, H. 1993. New research on poverty and malnutrition: What are the implications for poverty? In *Including the poor*, ed. M. Lipton and J. van der Gaag. Washington, D.C.: World Bank.

Alderman, H., and P. Gertler. 1989. The substitutability of public and private health care for the treatment of children in Pakistan. International Food Policy Research Institute, Washington, D.C., and The Rand Corporation. Mimeo.

Alvarez, M., and P. Perez. 1989. Developmental quotient in malnourished infants. In *Abstracts of Fourteenth Meeting of the International Congress of Nutrition*, 464. Seoul: Secretariat, Department of Food and Nutrition, Ewha Woman's University.

Annegers, J. F. 1973. Seasonal food shortages in West Africa. *Ecology of Food and Nutrition* 2: 251-257.

Arteaga, H. 1982. Obesity among schoolchildren of different economic levels in a developing country. *International Journal of Obesity* 6.

Ashworth, A., and D. J. Millward. 1986. Catch-up growth in children. *Nutrition Reviews* 44 (5): 157-164.

Aspelin, P. 1979. Food distribution and social bonding among the Mamainde of Mato Grosso, Brazil. *Journal of Anthropological Research* 35: 309-327.

Åstrand, I. 1967. Degree of strain during building work as related to individual aerobic capacity. *Ergonomics* 10: 293-303.

Barac-Nieto, M., G. B. Spurr, and J. C. Reina. 1984. Marginal malnutrition in school-aged Colombian boys: Body composition and maximal O_2 consumption. *American Journal of Clinical Nutrition* 39: 830-839.

Barnicot, N. A. 1964. Biological variation in modern populations. In *Human Biology*, ed. G. A. Harrison, J. S. Weiner, J. M. Tanner, and N. A. Barnicot, 189-291. Oxford, U.K.: Clarendon.

Barrett, D. E., M. Radke-Yarrow, and R. E. Klein. 1982. Chronic malnutrition and child behaviour: Effects of early caloric supplementation on social and emotional functioning at school age. *Developmental Psychology* 18: 541-556.

Basta, S. 1977. Nutrition and health in low-income areas of the third world. *Ecology of Food and Nutrition* 16: 105-126.

Beaton, G. H. 1985. The significance of adaptation in the definition of nutrient requirements and for nutrition policy. In *Nutritional adaptation in man*, ed. K. Blaxter and J. Waterlow, 219-232. London: Libbey.

———. 1989. Small but healthy? Are we asking the right question? *Human Organization* 48 (1): 31-37.

Beaton, G. H., and H. Ghassemi. 1982. Supplementary feeding programmes for young children in developing countries. *American Journal of Clinical Nutrition* 35: 864-916.

Behrman, J., and A. Deolalikar. 1988. Health and nutrition. In *Handbook of development economics*, vol. 1, ed. H. Chenery and T. N. Srinivasan. Amsterdam: North-Holland.

Behrman, J., and B. L. Wolfe. 1984. More evidence on nutritional demand. *Journal of Development Economics* 14 (1-2): 105-128.

Behrman, J. R. 1988a. *Nutrient intakes and income: Tightly wedded or loosely meshed?* Pew Memorial Trusts and Cornell Food and Nutrition Policy Program Lecture. Ithaca, N.Y., U.S.A.: Cornell University.

———. 1988b. Nutrition, health, birth order and seasonality: Intrahousehold allocation in rural India. *Journal of Development Economics* 28 (February): 43-63.

———. 1988c. Intrahousehold allocation of nutrients in rural India: Are boys favored? Do parents exhibit inequality aversion? *Oxford Economic Papers* 40 (March): 32-54.

———. 1990. The intrahousehold demand for nutrients in rural South India: Individual estimates, fixed effects and permanent income. *Journal of Human Resources* 25 (4): 665-696.

Belkenchir, D., Z. Belhocine, N. Ould-Ruis, A. Labara, and S. Kermani. 1985. Etat nutritionelle et diarrhée aigue du nourrisson. In *Les malnutritions dans les pays du tiers-monde: Abstracts of the Thirteenth International Congress of Nutrition*, ed. D. Lemonnier and Y. Inglebleek. Paris: Institut National de la Santé et de la Recherche Médicale.

Benedict, F. G., W. R. Miles, P. Roth, and H. M. Smith. 1919. *Human vitality and efficiency under prolonged restricted diet*. Washington, D.C.: Carnegie Press.

Benefice, E., S. Chevassus-Agnes, and H. Barral. 1984. Nutritional situation and seasonal variations for pastoralist populations of the Sahel (Senegalese Ferlo). *Ecology of Food and Nutrition* 14: 229-247.

Bentley, G. R. 1985. Hunter-gatherer energetics and fertility: A reassessment of the !Kung San. *Human Ecology* 13 (1): 79-109.

Bhanoji Rao, V. 1981. Measurement of deprivation and poverty based on the proportion spent on food. *World Development* 9 (4): 337-353.

Bhaskaram, P., R. Satyanarayana, J. S. Prasad, V. Jagadeesan, A. Naidu, and V. Reddy. 1980. Effect of growth retardation in early life on immunocompetence in later life. *Indian Journal of Medical Research* 72: 519-526.

Black, S. J., and D. Sanjur. 1980. Nutrition in Rio Piedras: A study of internal migration and maternal diets. *Ecology of Food and Nutrition* 10: 25-33.

Blaxter, K., and J. Waterlow, eds. 1985. *Nutritional adaptation in man.* London: Libbey.

Bleiburg, F. M., T. A. Brun, and S. Goiham. 1980. Duration of activities and energy expenditure of female farmers in dry and rainy seasons in Upper Volta. *British Journal of Nutrition* 43: 71.

Bogen, K., and R. Crittenden. 1987. Environment, economic development and the nutritional status of children in the southern highlands of Papua New Guinea in 1983. *Ecology of Food and Nutrition* 20: 29-49.

Bouchard, C., A. Tremblay, A. Nadeau, J. P. Despres, G. Theriault, M. R. Boulay, G. Lortie, C. Leblanc, and G. Fournier. 1989. Genetic effect in resting and exercise metabolic rates. *Metabolism* 38 (4): 364-370.

Bouis, H., and L. Haddad. 1988. Commercialization of agriculture in the southern Philippines. International Food Policy Research Institute, Washington, D.C. Mimeo.

————. 1990. *Effects of agricultural commercialization on land tenure, household resource allocation, and nutrition in the Philippines.* Research Report 79. Washington, D.C.: International Food Policy Research Institute.

Braun, J. von, and E. Kennedy. 1986. *Commercialization of subsistence agriculture: Income and nutritional effects in developing countries.* Working Papers on Commercialization of Agriculture and Nutrition No. 1. Washington, D.C.: International Food Policy Research Institute.

Braun, J. von, D. Hotchkiss, and M. Immink. 1989. *Nontraditional export crops in Guatemala: Effects on production, income, and nutrition.* Research Report 73. Washington, D.C.: International Food Policy Research Institute.

Briend, A. 1984. Feeding the fetus in the tropics: Rest is best. *Journal of Tropical Pediatrics* 30: 126-128.

Briscoe, J. 1979. The quantitative effect of infection on the use of food by children in poor countries. *American Journal of Clinical Nutrition* 32: 648-673.

Brooke, O. G. 1986. Energy needs during infancy. In *Energy and protein needs during infancy*, ed. S. J. Fomon and W. C. Heird. Orlando, Fla., U.S.A.: Academic Press.

Brooks, R. M., M. C. Latham, and D. W. T. Crompton. 1979. The relationship of nutrition and health to worker productivity in Kenya. *East African Medical Journal* 56: 413-421.

Brown, K., R. Black, and S. Becker. 1982. Seasonal changes in nutritional status and the prevalence of malnutrition in a longitudinal study of young children in rural Bangladesh. *American Journal of Clinical Nutrition* 36: 303-313.

Brown, K., R. Black, A. Robertson, and S. Becker. 1985. Effects of season and illness on the dietary intake of weanlings during longitudinal studies in rural Bangladesh. *American Journal of Clinical Nutrition* 41: 343-355.

Brozek, J. 1979. *Behavioral effects of energy and protein deficits.* NIH Publication No. 79-1906. Bethesda, Md., U.S.A.: National Institutes of Health.

Butz, W. P., J. P. Habicht, and J. DaVanzo. 1984. Environmental factors in the relationship between breast feeding and infant mortality: The role of sanitation and water in Malaysia. *Americal Journal of Epidemiology* 119(4): 516-525.

Buzina, R., C. J. Bates, J. van der Beek, G. Brubacher, R. K. Chandra, L. Hallberg, J. Heseker, W. Mertz, K. Pietrazik, E. Pollitt, A. Pradilla, H. H. Sandstead, W. Schalch, G. B. Spurr, and J. Westerhofer. 1989. Workshop on functional significance of mild-to-moderate malnutrition. *American Journal of Clinical Nutrition* 50: 172-176.

Campbell, D. J. 1984. Response to drought among farmers and herders in Southern Kajiado District, Kenya. *Human Ecology* 12 (1): 35-64.

_____. 1987. Strategies for coping with severe food deficits in north-eastern Africa. *Northeast African Studies* 9 (2): 43-54.

Campbell, D. J., and D. Trechter. 1982. Strategies for coping with food consumption shortage in the Mandara Mountains region of North Cameroon. *Social Science and Medicine* 16: 2117-2127.

Chaliha Kalita, M., and S. Seshadri. 1989. Anemia, undernutrition and productivity. In *Abstracts of Fourteenth Meeting of the International Congress of Nutrition*, 341. Seoul: Secretariat, Department of Food and Nutrition, Ewha Woman's University.

Chambers, R., R. Longhurst, and A. Pacey, eds. 1981. Seasonal dimensions to rural poverty. Totowa, N.J., U.S.A.: Allanheld, Osmun.

Chandra, R. 1981. Marginal malnutrition and immunocompetence. In *Nutrition in health and disease and international development*, ed. A. Harper and G. Davis. New York: Liss.

_____. 1991. Nutrition and immunity: Lessons from the past and new insights into the future. *American Journal of Clinical Nutrition* 53 (5): 1087-1101.

Chavez, A., and C. Martinez. 1982. *Growing up in a developing community*. Mexico City: Instituto Nacional de Nutrición.

Chen, L. C., A. K. M. Chowdhury, and S. L. Huffman. 1980. Anthropometric assessment of energy-protein malnutrition and subsequent risk of mortality among pre-school-aged children. *American Journal of Clinical Nutrition* 33: 1836-1845.

Chen, L. C., E. Huq, and S. D'Souza. 1981. Sex bias in the family allocation of food and health care in rural Bangladesh. *Population and Development Review* 1: 1.

Chitre, R., S. Deshpande, and S. N. Nimbalkar. 1983. The process of human adaptation in malnourished populations with special reference to tribals. Part 1: Food and nutrient intake of Mahadeo Koli from Khireshwar. *Indian Journal of Nutrition and Dietetics* 20: 46-55.

Chung, A. W., and B. Viscorova. 1948. The effect of early oral feeding versus early starvation on the course of infant diarrhoea. *Journal of Pediatrics* 33: 14.

Clark, C., and M. Haswell. 1970. *The economics of subsistence agriculture*. London: Macmillan.

Clark, W. 1980. The rural to urban nutritional gradient: Application and interpretation in a developing nation and urban situation. *Social Science and Medicine* 14D: 31-36.

Clay, E. 1981. Seasonal patterns of agricultural employment in Bangladesh. In *Seasonal dimensions to rural poverty*, ed. R. Chambers, R. Longhurst, and A. Pacey, 92-101. Totowa, N.J., U.S.A.: Allanheld, Osmun.

Cole, T. J., J. C. Gilson, and C. H. Olsen. 1974. Bronchitis, smoking, and obesity in an English and a Danish town: Male deaths after a 10-year follow-up. Bulletin of the Physiology-Pathology of Respiration 10 (5): 657-679.

Commission on Health Research for Development. 1990. *Health research: Essential link to equity in development.* New York: Oxford University Press.

Cornu, A., O. Pondi Njiki, and T. Agbor Egbe. 1985. Anémie et malnutrition chez l'enfant de la province du Nord-Cameroun. In *Les malnutritions dans les pays du tiers-monde: Abstracts of the Thirteenth International Congress of Nutrition,* ed. D. Lemonnier and Y. Inglebleek. Paris: Institut National de la Santé et de la Recherche Médicale.

Crabbe, G. [1783] 1987. The Village. In *George Crabbe: The complete poetical works.* Oxford, U.K.: Clarendon.

Crittenden, R., and J. Baines. 1985. Assessments of the nutritional status of children on the Nembi Plateau in 1978 and 1980. *Ecology of Food and Nutrition* 17: 131-147.

_____. 1986. The seasonal factors influencing child nutrition on the Nembi Plateau, Papua New Guinea. *Human Ecology* 14 (2): 191-223.

Dasgupta, P., and D. Ray. 1986. Adapting to undernourishment: The clinical evidence and its implications. Economic Theory Discussion Paper. Department of Applied Economics, Cambridge University, Cambridge, U.K. Mimeo.

Datta, G., and J. Meerman. 1980. *Household income and household income per capita in welfare comparisons.* World Bank Staff Working Paper No. 378. Washington, D.C.: World Bank.

Davidson, S., R. Passmore, J. F. Brock, and A. S. Truswell. 1975. *Human nutrition and dietetics.* 6th ed. Edinburgh: Churchill Livingstone.

Davies, D. P. 1988. The importance of genetic influences on growth in early childhood, with particular reference to children of Asiatic region. In *Linear growth retardation in less developed countries,* ed. J. C. Waterlow. Nestlé Nutrition Workshop Series, vol. 14. Vevey, Switzerland: Raven Press.

Day, J., A. Bailey, and D. Robinson. 1979. Biological variations associated with change in lifestyle among the pastoral and nomadic tribes of East Africa. *Annals of Human Biology* 6 (1): 29-39.

de Almeida, M. D., and J. E. Thomas. 1989. Migration and changing food habits. In *Abstracts of Fourteenth Meeting of the International Congress of Nutrition,* 461. Seoul: Secretariat, Department of Food and Nutrition, Ewha Woman's University.

Deaton, A., J. Ruiz-Castillo, and D. Thomas. 1984. The influence of household composition on household expenditure patterns: Theory and Spanish evidence. Princeton University, Princeton, N.J., U.S.A. Mimeo.

de Chavez, M. M., P. Arroyo, S. E. Perez Gil, M. Hernandez, S. E. Quiroz, M. Rodriguez, M. P. de Hermelo, and A. Chavez. 1974. The epidemiology of good nutrition in a population with a high prevalence of malnutrition. *Ecology of Food and Nutrition* 3: 223-230.

Dennett, C., and J. Connell. 1988. Acculturation and health in the highlands of Papua New Guinea. *Current Anthropology* 29 (2): 273-281.

Desai, I. D., C. Waddell, S. Dutra, S. Dutra de Oliveria, E. Duarte, M. L. Robazzi, L. S. Cevallos Romero, M. I. Desai, F. L. Vichi, R. B. Bradfield, and J. E. Dutra de Oliveria. 1984. Marginal malnutrition and reduced physical work capacity of migrant adolescent boys in southern Brazil. *American Journal of Clinical Nutrition* 40: 135-145.

DeWatt, K. 1983. Income and dietary adequacy in an agricultural community. *Social Science and Medicine* 17 (23): 1877-1886.

Diaz, E., G. Goldberg, M. Taylor, J. Savage, D. Sellen, W. Coward, and A. Prentice. 1989. Effects of dietary supplementation on work performance in Gambian labourers. In *Abstracts of Fourteenth Meeting of the International Congress of Nutrition.* Seoul: Secretariat, Department of Food and Nutrition, Ewha Woman's University.

Dirks, R. 1980. Social responses during severe food shortage and famine. *Current Anthropology* 21 (1): 21-44.

Drèze, J., and A. K. Sen. 1989. *Hunger and public action.* Oxford, U.K.: Clarendon.

Dugdale, A. E., and P. R. Payne. 1987. A model of seasonal changes in energy balance. *Ecology of Food and Nutrition* 19: 231-245.

Dunn Nutrition Unit. 1986. *Cambridge, U.K., and Keneba, The Gambia, 1982-85.* Cambridge, U.K.: Dunn.

Durnin, J. V. G. A. 1988. Energy requirements of pregnancy and lactation. In *Proceedings of the meeting of the International Dietary Energy Consultation,* ed. B. Schurch and N. S. Scrimshaw, 135-152. Lausanne, Switzerland: Nestlé Foundation.

Durnin, J. V. G. A., J. Womersley, and R. Campbell. 1976. A study of energy balance on ten male Ethiopian labourers on low energy intakes. *Nutrition Society Symposium Proceedings* 35: 145.

Durnin, J. V. G. A., F. M. McKillon, S. Grant, and G. L. Fitzgerald. 1985. Is nutritional status endangered by virtually no extra intake in pregnancy? *Lancet* 2: 823.

Dyson, T., and N. Crook. 1981. Causes of seasonal fluctuation in vital events. In *Seasonal dimensions to rural poverty*, ed. R. Chambers, R. Longhurst, and A. Pacey, 135-154. Totowa, N.J., U.S.A.: Allanheld, Osmun.

Edirisinghe N., and T. Poleman, 1983. Behavioural thresholds as indicators of perceived dietary adequacy or inadequacy. Agricultural Economics Research Paper No. 83-24. Cornell/International Agricultural Economics Study. Cornell University, Ithaca, N.Y. Mimeo.

Edmundson, W. 1979. Individual variations in basal metabolic rate and mechanical work efficiency in East Java. *Ecology of Food and Nutrition* 8: 189-195.

Edmundson, W., and S. Edmundson. 1989. Food intake and work allocation of male and female farmers in an impoverished Indian village. *British Journal of Nutrition* 60: 433-439.

Edmundson, W., and P. Sukhatme. 1990. Food and work: Poverty and hunger? *Economic Development and Cultural Change* 38 (2): 263-280.

Eveleth, P. B. 1985. Nutritional implications of differences in adolescent growth and maturation and in adult body size. In *Nutritional adaptation in man*, ed. K. Blaxter and J. Waterlow, 31-43. London: Libbey.

Eveleth, P. B., and J. M. Tanner. 1976. *Worldwide variation in human growth*. Cambridge, U.K.: Cambridge University Press.

FAO/WHO (Food and Agriculture Organization of the United Nations/World Health Organization). 1973. *Energy and protein requirements*. Geneva: WHO.

FAO/WHO/UNU (Food and Agriculture Organization of the United Nations/World Health Organization/United Nations University). 1985. *Energy and protein requirements*. Geneva: WHO.

Farhat Sultana. 1989. Mothers' nutritional/health status and its impact on their child care activities. In *Abstracts of Fourteenth Meeting of the International Congress of Nutrition*, 224. Seoul: Secretariat, Department of Food and Nutrition, Ewha Woman's University.

Ferro-Luzzi, A. 1985. Work capacity and productivity in long-term adaptation to low energy intakes. In *Nutritional adaptation in man*, ed. K. Blaxter and J. Waterlow, 61-68. London: Libbey.

Ferro-Luzzi, A., G. Pastore, and S. Sette. 1988. Seasonality in energy metabolism. In *Chronic energy deficiency: Consequences and related issues*, ed. B. Schurch and N. Scrimshaw, 37-58. Lausanne, Switzerland: Nestlé Foundation.

Firth, Raymond. 1959. *Social change in Tikopia: Re-study of a Polynesian community after a generation.* New York: Macmillan.

Florencio, C. A. 1989. Nutrient intakes and school performance of Filipino children. In *Abstracts of Fourteenth Meeting of the International Congress of Nutrition*, 339. Seoul: Secretariat, Department of Food and Nutrition, Ewha Woman's University.

Fomon, S.J., and W. C. Heird, eds. 1986. *Energy and protein needs during infancy.* Orlando, Fla., U.S.A.: Academic Press.

Galvin, K. 1985. Food procurement, diet, activities and nutrition of Ngisonyoka, Turkana pastoralists in an ecological and social context. Ph.D. diss., State University of New York, Binghamton, N.Y., U.S.A.

Garby, L. 1987. Metabolic adaptation to decrease in energy intake due to changes in the energy cost of low-energy expenditure regimen. Report to Food and Agriculture Organization of the United Nations. Mimeo.

Geissler, C. A., and M. S. H. Aldouri. 1985. Racial differences in the energy cost of standardized activities. *Annals of Nutrition and Metabolism* 29: 40-47.

Girardier, L., and M. J. Stock. 1983. *Mammalian thermogenesis.* London: Chapman and Hall.

Glewwe, P., and J. van der Gaag. 1988. *Confronting poverty in developing countries.* Living Standards Measurement Study Working Paper No. 48. Washington, D.C.: World Bank.

Gopalan, C. 1983. Measurement of undernutrition: Biological considerations. *Economic and Political Weekly* 18 (15): 591-595.

Gould, S. J., and R. C. Lewontin. 1979. The spandrels of San Marco and the Panglossian paradigm: A critique of the adaptationist programme. Proceedings of the Royal Society of London B205: 581-598.

Graham, G., H. Creed, W. MacLean, C. Kallman, J. Rabold, and D. Mellits. 1981. Determinants of growth among poor children: Nutrient intake-achieved growth relationships. *American Journal of Clinical Nutrition* 34: 539-554.

Grande, F. 1984. Body weight, composition and energy balance. *Nutrition Reviews.*

Grivetti, L. E. 1978. Nutritional success in a semi-arid land: Examination of Tswana agro-pastoralists of the eastern Kalahari, Botswana. *American Journal of Clinical Nutrition* 31: 1204-1220.

Gross, D., and B. Underwood. 1971. Technological change and calorie costs: Sisal agriculture in NE Brazil. *American Anthropologist* 73: 725-740.

Guldan, G. S., M. F. Zeitlin, C. M. Super, and A. Beiser. 1989. Maternal education and child feeding practices in rural Bangladesh. In *Abstracts of Fourteenth Meeting of the International Congress of Nutrition*, 462. Seoul: Secretariat, Department of Food and Nutrition, Ewha Woman's University.

Haas, J. 1983. Nutrition and high altitude adaptation: An example of human adaptability in a multistress environment. In *Rethinking human adaptation: Biological and cultural models*, ed. R. Dyson-Hudson and M. Little, 41-56. Boulder, Colo., U.S.A.: Westview Press.

Harper, A., and G. Davis, eds. 1981. *Nutrition in health and disease and international development*. New York: Liss.

Harriss, B. 1986. *The intrafamily distribution of hunger in South Asia*. Helsinki: WIDER.

Hart, T. B., and J. A. Hart. 1986. The ecological basis of hunter-gatherer subsistence in African rain forests: The Mbuti of Eastern Zaire. *Human Ecology* 14 (1): 29-55.

Henry, C. J. K., and D. G. Rees. 1989. A preliminary analysis of BMR and race. In *Comparative nutrition*, ed. K. Blaxter and I. MacDonald, 149-159. London: Libbey.

Heywood, P. F. 1982. The functional significance of malnutrition: Growth and prospective risk of death in the highlands of Papua New Guinea. *Journal of Food and Nutrition* 39 (1): 13-19.

————. 1986. *Nutritional status as a risk factor for mortality in children in the highlands of Papua New Guinea: Proceedings of the Thirteenth International Congress of Nutrition*. London: Libbey.

Hipsley, E. 1969. *Metabolic rates in New Guineans*. Technical Paper No. 162. Noumea: South Pacific Commission.

Hopper, W. D. 1955. Seasonal labour cycles in an Eastern Uttar Pradesh village. *The Eastern Anthropologist* 8 (3 and 4).

Hoyle, B., M. Yunus, and L. C. Chen. 1980. Breast feeding and food intake among children with acute diarrhoeal disease. *American Journal of Clinical Nutrition* 33: 2365.

Huffman, S. L. 1983. Maternal and child nutritional status: Its association with the risk of pregnancy. *Social Science and Medicine* 17 (20): 1529-1540.

Hull, D. 1979. Migration, adaptation and illness: A review. *Social Science and Medicine* 13A: 25-36.

Hurtado, A. M., K. Hawkes, K. Hill, and H. Kaplan. 1985. Female subsistence strategies among Ache hunter-gatherers of eastern Paraguay. *Human Ecology* 13 (1): 1-28.

Hytten, F. E., and I. Leitch. 1971. *The physiology of human pregnancy.* Oxford: Blackwell.

ICN (International Congress of Nutrition). 1989. *Abstracts of Fourteenth Meeting of the International Congress of Nutrition.* Seoul: Secretariat, Department of Food and Nutrition, Ewha Woman's University.

Immink, M. D. C., F. E. Viteri, F. Flores, and B. Torún. 1984. Microeconomic consequences of energy deficiency in rural populations in developing countries. In *Energy intake and activity,* ed. E. Pollitt and P. Amante. New York: Alan R. Liss.

James, W. P. T. 1985. Appetite control and other mechanisms of weight homeostasis. In *Nutritional adaptation in man,* ed. K. Blaxter and J. Waterlow. London: Libbey.

Jodha, N. 1975. Famine and famine policies: Some empirical evidence. *Economic and Political Weekly* 41 (10): 1609-1623.

Kashiwazaki, H. 1983. Agricultural practices and household organization in a Japanese pioneer community of lowland Bolivia. *Human Ecology* 11 (3): 283-319.

Keller, W., and C. Fillmore. 1983. Prevalence of protein-energy malnutrition. *World Health Statistical Quarterly* 36: 128-167.

Keusch, G. T., and M. J. G. Farthing. 1986. Nutrition and infection. *Annual Reviews of Nutrition* 6: 131-154.

Keys, A. 1980. Overweight, obesity, coronary disease and mortality. *Nutrition Reviews* 38: 297-306.

Keys, A., J. Brozek, A. Henschel, O. Mickelson, and H. L. Taylor. 1950. *The biology of human starvation.* Minneapolis, Minn., U.S.A.: University of Minnesota Press.

Kielmann, A., and C. McCord. 1978. Weight-for-age as an index of risk of death in children. *Lancet* (1): 1247-1250.

Kielmann, A. A., C. DeSweemer, W. Blot, I.S. Uberoi, A. Douglas-Robertson, and C. E. Taylor. 1978. Impact of child growth and nutrition on psychomotor development. In *Child and maternal health services in rural India: The Narangwal experiment,* vol. 1, ed. A. Kielmann et al. Washington, D.C.: World Bank.

Koster, F., D. Palmer, J. Chakraborty, T. Jackson, and P. Gurlin. 1987. Cellular immune competence and diarrhoeal morbidity in malnourished Bangladesh children: A prospective field study. *American Journal of Clinical Nutrition* 46: 115-120.

Lawrence, M., and R. G. Whitehead. 1989. Energy utilization in undernourished lactating women. In *Abstracts of Fourteenth Meeting of the International Congress of Nutrition*, 179. Seoul: Secretariat, Department of Food and Nutrition, Ewha Woman's University.

Lawrence, M., F. McKillop, and J. Durnin. 1989. The composition of weight gained during pregnancy and its relationship to birthweight. In *Annual Report 1988*. Lausanne, Switzerland: Nestlé Foundation.

Lawrence, M., J. Singh, F. Lawrence, and R. G. Whitehead. 1985. The energy cost of common daily activities in African women: Increased expenditure in pregnancy? *American Journal of Clinical Nutrition* 42: 753-763.

Lawrence, M., W. A. Coward, F. Lawrence, T. J. Cole, and R. G. Whitehead. 1987. Fat gain during pregnancy in rural African women: The effect of season and dietary status. *American Journal of Clinical Nutrition* 45: 1442-1450.

Lazear, E., and R. Michael. 1980. Family size and the distribution of real per capita income. *American Economic Review* 70 (1): 91-107.

Lechtig, A., C. Yarborough, H. Delgado, J-P. Habicht, R. Martorell, and R. Klein. 1975. Influence of maternal nutrition on birth weight. *American Journal of Clinical Nutrition* 28: 1223-1237.

Lee, D. H. K. 1977. *Climate and economic development in the tropics.* New York: Harper and Brothers.

Lee, R. B. 1973. Mongongo: The ethnography of a major wild food resource. *Ecology of Food and Nutrition* 2: 307-313.

Lepowsky, M. A. 1985. Food taboos, malaria and dietary change: Infant feeding and cultural adaptation on a Papua New Guinea island. *Ecology of Food and Nutrition* 16: 105-126.

Lipton, M. 1983a. *Poverty, undernutrition and hunger.* World Bank Staff Working Paper No. 597. Washington, D.C.: World Bank.

———. 1983b. *Labour and poverty.* World Bank Staff Working Paper No. 616. Washington, D.C.: World Bank.

———. 1983c. *Demography and poverty.* World Bank Staff Working Paper No. 623. Washington, D.C.: World Bank.

———. 1985a. A case for democracy in less developed countries. In *Economy and Democracy*, ed. R. C. O. Matthews. London: Macmillan.

_____. 1985b. *Land assets and rural poverty.* World Bank Staff Working Paper No. 744. Washington, D.C.: World Bank.

_____. 1989. *Attacking undernutrition and poverty: Some issues of adaptation and sustainability.* Pew/Cornell Lectures on Food and Nutrition Policy. Ithaca, N.Y., U.S.A.: Cornell Food and Nutrition Policy Program.

Longhurst, R. 1982. Review of twelve national nutrition surveys. Food Policy and Nutrition Division, Food and Agriculture Organization of the United Nations, Rome. Mimeo.

_____. 1986. Food strategies in response to seasonality and famine. *IDS Bulletin* 17 (3): 27-35.

Longhurst, R., and P. Payne. 1981. Seasonal aspects of nutrition. In *Seasonal dimensions to rural poverty,* ed. R. Chambers, R. Longhurst, and A. Pacey, 45-52. Totowa, N.J., U.S.A.: Allanheld, Osmun.

Maclachlan, M. D. 1983. *Why they did not starve: Biocultural adaption in a South Indian village.* Philadelphia, Pa., U.S.A.: Institute of Human Issues.

Malcolm, L. A. 1974. Protein energy malnutrition and growth. In *Human Growth,* vol. 3, *Neurobiology and Nutrition,* ed. F. Falkner and J. M. Tanner, 361-372. London: Bailliere Tindall.

Martorell, R. 1982. Genetics, environment and growth in the assessment of nutritional status. In *Genetic factors in nutrition,* ed. A. Velazquez and H. Bourges, 373-391. Orlando, Fla., U.S.A.: Academic Press.

_____. 1985. Child growth retardation: A discussion of its causes and its relationship to health. In *Nutritional adaptation in man,* ed. K. Blaxter and J. Waterlow, 13-29. London: Libbey.

Martorell, R., and T. J. Ho. 1984. Malnutrition, morbidity and mortality. *Population and Development Review* 10 (Supplement).

Martorell, R., R. E. Klein, and H. Delgado. 1980. Improved nutrition and its effects on anthropometric indicators of nutritional status. *Nutrition Reports International* 21: 219-230.

Mason, E. D., M. Jacob, and V. Balakrishnan. 1964. Racial group differences in the basal metabolism and body composition of Indian and European women in Bombay. *Human Biology* 36: 374-396.

Maxwell, P., ed. 1988. Cash crops in developing countries. *Bulletin of the Institute of Development Studies* 19 (2).

McGregor, I.A., A. K. Rahman, B. Thompson, W. Z. Billewicz, and A. M. Thomson. 1968. The growth of young children in a Gambian village. *Transactions of the Royal Society of Tropical Medicine and Hygiene* 62 (3): 341-352.

McNeill, G. 1986. Patterns of adult energy nutrition in a South Indian village, Ph.D. diss., University of London, London.

McNeill, G., and P. R. Payne. 1985. Energy expenditure of pregnant and lactating women. *Lancet* 2: 1237.

McNeill, G., J. P. W. Rivers, P. R. Payne, J. J. de Britto, and R. Abel. 1987. Basal metabolic rate of Indian men: No evidence of metabolic adaptation to a low plane of nutrition. *Human Nutrition: Clinical Nutrition* 41C: 473-483.

Merimée, T.J., J. Zarf, B. Hewlett, and L. L. Sforza Cavalli. 1987. Insulin-like growth factors in Pygmies: The role of puberty in determining final stature. *New England Journal of Medicine* 316: 906-911.

Messer, E. 1986. The "small but healthy" hypothesis: Historical, political and ecological influences on nutritional standards. *Human Ecology* 14 (1): 57-75.

Michael, E. D., K. E. Hutton, and S. M. Horvath. 1961. Cardiorespiratory responses during prolonged exercise. *Journal of Applied Physiology* 16: 997-1000.

Miller, D. S. 1982. Factors affecting energy expenditure. *Proceedings of the Nutritional Society* 41: 193-201.

Milligan, L. P., and M. Summers. 1986. The biological basis of maintenance and its relevance to assessing responses to nutrients. *Proceedings of the Nutritional Society* 45: 185.

Millman, S. R., and R. S. Chen. 1991. *Measurement of hunger: Defining thresholds.* Brown University Research Report RR-91-6. Providence, R.I., U.S.A.: World Hunger Program.

Molla, A., A. M. Molla, S. A. Sarker, M. Khatoon, and M. Rahaman. 1983. Effects of acute diarrhoea on absorption of micronutrients during disease and after recovery. In *Diarrhoea and malnutrition*, ed. L. C. Chen and N. S. Scrimshaw, 143-154. New York and London: Plenum.

Morris, M. D. 1974. What is a famine? *Economic and Political Weekly*, November 2: 1855-1864.

Mosher, S. W. 1979. Birth seasonality among peasant cultivators: The interrelationship of workload, diet and fertility. *Human Ecology* 7 (2): 151-181.

Mo-Suwan, L. 1989. Maternal nutrition and the outcome of pregnancy in the rural area of southern Thailand. In *Abstracts of Fourteenth Meeting of the International Congress of Nutrition*, 601. Seoul: Secretariat, Department of Food and Nutrition, Ewha Woman's University.

Murray, M., A. Murray, N. Murray, and M. Murray. 1978. Diet and cerebral malaria: The effect of famine and refeeding. *American Journal of Clinical Nutrition* 31: 57-61.

Nestlé Foundation. 1988. *Annual report 1988.* Lausanne, Switzerland.

Neumann, C. G., N. O. Bwibo, and M. Sigman. 1993. Diet quantity and quality: Functional effects on rural Kenyan families, 1989-1992. Final report to Office of Nutrition, U.S. Agency for International Development, Washington, D.C.

Neumann, C. G., G. Beaton, E. Carter, M. Paolisso, G. Gardner, and N. O. Bwibo. 1989. Effect of reduced food intake on resting metabolic rate in rural Kenyan men. In *Abstracts of Fourteenth Meeting of the International Congress of Nutrition.* Seoul: Secretariat, Department of Food and Nutrition, Ewha Woman's University.

Nicol, B. M., and P. G. Phillips. 1976. The utilization of dietary protein by Nigerian men. *British Journal of Nutrition* 36: 337-351.

Nieves, I., and P. L. Engle. 1989. Maternal food management and intrahousehold food distribution in Guatemala. In *Abstracts of Fourteenth Meeting of the International Congress of Nutrition,* 179. Seoul: Secretariat, Department of Food and Nutrition, Ewha Woman's University.

Norgan, N., A. Ferro-Luzzi, and J. Durnin. 1982. The body composition of New Guinean adults in contrasting environments. *Annals of Human Biology* 9: 343-353.

Ohtsuka, R., T. Inaoka, T. Kawabe, T. Suzuki, T. Hongo, and T. Akimichi. 1985. Diversity and change of food consumption and nutrient intake among the Gidra in lowland Papua. *Ecology of Food and Nutrition* 16: 339-350.

Okeke, E. C., D. O. Nnanyelugo, and E. Ngwu. 1983. Prevalence of obesity in adults in Anambra State, Nigeria. *Growth* 47 (3): 263-271.

Osmani, S. 1988. Nutrition and the economics of food: Implications of some recent controversies. In *Entitlement and well-being,* vol. 1 of *The political economy of hunger,* ed. J. Drèze and A. K. Sen. Oxford, U.K.: Clarendon Press.

————. 1990. Economics of food and nutrition: Some controversies. In *Entitlement and well-being,* vol. 1 of *The political economy of hunger,* ed. J. Drèze and A. K. Sen. Oxford, U.K.: Clarendon Press.

Pagezy, H. 1984. Seasonal hunger as experienced by the Oto and the Twa women of a Ntomba village in the equatorial forest (Lake Tumba, Zaire). *Ecology of Food and Nutrition* 15: 13-27.

Pariza, M. W. 1987. Dietary fat, calorie restriction, ad libitum feeding and cancer risk. *Nutrition Reviews* 45 (1): 1-7.

Payne, P. R. 1986. Appropriate indicators for project design and evaluation. In *Food aid and the well-being of children in the developing world.* New York: UNICEF/World Food Programme.

Payne, P. R., and A. Dugdale. 1977. A model for the prediction of energy balance and body weight. *Annals of Human Biology* 4 (6): 525-536.

Pelletier, David. L. 1991. *Relationships between child anthropometry and mortality in developing countries: Implications for policy, programs, and future research.* Monograph 12. Ithaca, N.Y., U.S.A.: Cornell Food and Nutrition Policy Program.

Pelto, G. H., L. H. Allen, and A. Chavez. 1989. Household environment, caregiving and nutrition of children: Overview, with a case from highland Mexico. In *Abstracts of Fourteenth Meeting of the International Congress of Nutrition,* 221. Seoul: Secretariat, Department of Food and Nutrition, Ewha Woman's University.

Petrasek, R. 1978. Influence of climatic conditions on energy and nutrient requirements. *Progress in Food and Nutrition Science* 2 (11/12).

Pimental, N. A., and K. B. Pandolf. 1979. Energy expenditure while standing or walking slowly uphill or downhill with loads. *Ergonomics* 22 (8): 963-973.

Pingale, U. 1975. Some studies in two tribal groups of central India: Dietary intake and nutritional status. *Plant Foods for Man* 1: 185-194.

Poehlman, E. T., and M. S. Horton. 1989. The impact of food intake and exercise on energy expenditure. *Nutrition Reviews* 47 (5): 129-137.

Pollitt, E. 1990. *Malnutrition and infection in the classroom.* Paris: UNICEF.

Pollitt, E., and P. Amante. 1984. *Energy intake and activity.* New York: Alan Liss.

Pollitt, E., K. S. Gorman, P. L. Engle, R. Martorell, and J. Rivera. 1993. Early supplementary feeding and cognition: Effects over two decades. *Monographs of the Society for Research in Child Development,* vol. 58, no. 7. Chicago, Ill., U.S.A.: University of Chicago Press.

Pongpaew, P., F.-P. Schelp, N. Vudhivai, V. Supawan, and P. Migasena. 1988. Alpha-2 macroglobulin, 3-methylhistadine and other biochemical parameters in preschool children of marginal nutritional status: Some evidence of an adaptation process in sub-clinical PEM. *Nutrition Research* 8: 1213-1221.

Prentice, A. M., and A. Prentice. 1988. Energy costs of lactation. *Annual Reviews of Nutrition* 8: 63-79.

Prentice, A. M., S. B. Roberts, A. Prentice, A. A. Paul, M. Watkinson, A. Watkinson, and R. G. Whitehead. 1983a. Dietary supplementation of lactating Gambian women: Effect on breastmilk output and quality. *Human Nutrition: Clinical Nutrition* 37C: 53-64.

Prentice, A. M., R. G. Whitehead, M. Watkinson, W. H. Lamb, and T. J. Cole. 1983b. Pre-natal dietary supplementation of African women and birthweight. *Lancet* 1: 489-492.

Prentice, A., H. Davies, A. Black, J. Ashford, W. Coward, P. Murgatroyd, G. Goldberg, M. Sawyer, and R. Whitehead. 1985. Unexpectedly low levels of energy expenditure in healthy women. *Lancet* 22 (June): 1419-1422.

Prindle, P. M. 1979. Peasant society and famine: A Nepalese example. *Ethnology* 18 (1).

Pryer, J. 1990. Socioeconomic and environmental aspects of undernutrition and ill health in an urban slum in Bangladesh. Ph.D. thesis, London University, London.

Quandt, S. A. 1984. Nutritional thriftiness and human reproduction: Beyond the critical body composition hypothesis. *Social Science and Medicine* 19 (2): 177-182.

Quenouille, M. H., A. W. Boyne, W. B. Fisher, and I. Leitch. 1951. *Statistical studies of recorded energy expenditure of man, Part 1: Basal metabolism related to sex, stature, age, climate and race*. Technical Communication No. 17. Bucksburn, Scotland: Commonwealth Bureau of Animal Nutrition.

Rabiee, F., and C. Geissler. 1989. Maternal work and child nutrition in Iran. In *Abstracts of Fourteenth Meeting of the International Congress of Nutrition*, 226. Seoul: Secretariat, Department of Food and Nutrition, Ewha Woman's University.

Reddy, V., V. Jagadeesan, N. Ragharomalu, C. Bhaskaram, and S. Srikantia. 1976. Functional significance of growth retardation in malnutrition. *American Journal of Clinical Nutrition* 2A.

Riley, R. A. 1979. A dietary survey of downward Indian migrants and long-term coastal residents living in southern coastal Peru. *Archivos Latinoamericanos de Nutrición* 29 (1): 69-99.

Riumallo, J. A., and F. Monckeberg. 1983. Nutrition recovery centers: The Chilean experience. In *Nutrition intervention strategies in national development*, ed. B. Underwood. New York: Academic Press.

Roberts, D. 1985. Genetics and nutritional adaptation. In *Nutritional adaptation in man*, ed. K. Blaxter and J. Waterlow, 45-59. London: Libbey.

Robson, J., and G. Wadsworth. 1977. The health and nutritional status of primitive populations. *Ecology of Food and Nutrition* 6: 187-202.

Rosenzweig, M. R. 1988. Risk, implicit contracts and the family in rural areas of low-income countries. *The Economic Journal* 98 (December): 1148-1170.

Rosenzweig, M. R., and K. I. Wolpin. 1985. Specific experience, household structure and intergenerational transfers: Farm family land and labour arrangements in developing countries. *American Economic Review* 100 (Supplement).

Rosetta, L. 1986. Sex differences in seasonal variations of the nutritional status of Serere adults in Senegal. *Ecology of Food and Nutrition* 18: 231-244.

Ross, C., and Minkowsky, J. 1983. Social epidemiology of overweight. *Journal of Health and Social Behavior* 24.

Rothwell, N., and M. Stock. 1979. A note on brown adipose tissue in diet-induced thermogenesis. *Nature* 281: 31-35.

Rowland, M. G. M., A. Paul, A. M. Prentice, E. Muller, M. Hutton, and R. G. Whitehead. 1981. Seasonality and growth of infants in a Gambian village. In *Seasonal Dimensions to Rural Poverty*, ed. R. Chambers, R. Longhurst, and A. Pacey. Totowa, N.J., U.S.A.: Allanheld, Osmun.

Sambrani, S., and K. Pichcholiya. 1975. *An enquiry into rural poverty and unemployment*. Ahmedabad, India: Indian Institute of Management.

Satyanarayana, K., and M. Someshwar Rao. 1989. Nutrition and work performance: Studies carried out in India. In *Abstracts of Fourteenth Meeting of the International Congress of Nutrition*, 98-99. Seoul: Secretariat, Department of Food and Nutrition, Ewha Woman's University.

Satyanarayana, K., A. Nadamuni Naidu, and B. S. Narasinga Rao. 1979. Nutritional deprivation in childhood and the body size, activity and physical work capacity of young boys. *American Journal of Clinical Nutrition* 32: 1769-1775.

Satyanarayana, K., A. Nadamuni Naidu, B. Chatterjee, and B. Narasinga Rao. 1977. Body size and work output. *American Journal of Clinical Nutrition* 30: 322-325.

Schnetz, M., S. Egoramaiphol, and C. Leitzmann. 1984. Migration and nutrition in Thailand. *Ecology of Food and Nutrition* 15: 89-107.

Schofield, S. 1974. Seasonal factors affecting nutrition in different age groups and especially pre-school children. *Journal of Development Studies* 11 (1): 22-40.

————. 1979. *Development and the problems of village nutrition.* Sussex, U.K.: Croom Helm for Institute of Development Studies.

Schultze, K. 1986. A model of the variability in metabolic rate of neonates. In *Energy and protein needs during infancy,* ed. S. J. Fomon and W. C. Heird. Orlando, Fla., U.S.A.: Academic Press.

Seckler, D. 1980. Malnutrition: An intellectual odyssey. *Journal of the Western Agricultural Economics Association* (December).

————. 1985. Malnutrition: Definition, incidence, and effect on growth. *Growth Genetics and Hormones* 1: 7-8.

Seckler, D., and R. A. Young. 1978. Economic and policy implications of the 160-acre limitation in federal reclamation law. *American Journal of Agricultural Economics* (November).

Sen, A. K. 1981. *Poverty and famines.* Oxford, U.K.: Clarendon.

————. 1984. Rights and capabilities. In *Resources, values and development.* Oxford, U.K.: Blackwell.

Shah, A. 1968. Changes in the Indian family. *Economic and Political Weekly* 3 (1-2), Annual Number.

————. 1979. Household dimensions of the family in India. Berkeley, Calif. U.S.A.: University of California.

Shah, C. H. 1983. Food preferences and nutrition: A perspective on poverty. Presidential address, Indian Society of Agricultural Economics, Bangalore, India.

Shekar, M., J. P. Habicht, and M. C. Latham. 1989. Positive and negative deviance in a developing country: Is positive deviance in growth simply a mirror image of negative deviance? In *Abstracts of Fourteenth Meeting of the International Congress of Nutrition.* Seoul: Secretariat, Department of Food and Nutrition, Ewha Woman's University.

Shetty, P. S. 1984. Adaptive changes in basal metabolic rate and lean body mass in chronic undernutrition. *Human Nutrition: Clinical Nutrition* 38C: 443-451.

Shetty, P. S., A. V. Kurpad, K. N. Kulkarni, and M. Vaz. 1987. Thermogenic responses to norepinephrine in chronic energy deficiency. In *Annual Report 1988.* Lausanne, Switzerland: Nestlé Foundation.

Simmonds, N. 1981. *Principles of crop improvement.* New York: Longman.

Smith, E. A. 1979. Human adaptation and energetic efficiency. *Human Ecology* 7 (1): 53-74.

Sommers, A., and M. S. Lowenstein. 1975. Nutritional status and mortality: A prospective validation of the QUAC stick. *American Journal of Clinical Nutrition* 28: 287.

Spurr, G. B. 1984. Physical activity, nutritional status and physical work capacity in relation to agricultural productivity. In *Energy intake and activity*, ed. E. Pollitt and M. Amante. New York: A. R. Liss.

_____. 1986. Marginal malnutrition in school-aged Colombian boys: Body size and energy costs of walking and light load carrying. *Human Nutrition: Clinical Nutrition* 40C: 409-419.

_____. 1987. Marginal malnutrition in school-aged Colombian girls: Dietary intervention and daily energy expenditure. *Human Nutrition: Clinical Nutrition* 41C: 93-104.

Spurr, G. B., and J. C. Reina. 1989. Maximum oxygen consumption in marginally malnourished Colombian boys and girls 6-16 years of age. *American Journal of Human Biology* (1): 11-19.

Spurr, G. B., J. Reina, H. W. Dahners, and M. Barac-Nieto. 1983. Marginal malnutrition in school-aged Colombian boys: Functional consequences in maximum exercise. *American Journal of Clinical Nutrition* 37: 834-847.

_____. 1986. Marginal malnutrition in school-aged Colombian boys: Metabolic rates and estimated daily energy expenditure. *American Journal of Clinical Nutrition* 44: 113-126.

Stein, Z., and M. Susser. 1975. The Dutch famine, 1944-45, and the reproductive process, Part I. *Pediatric Research* 9.

Stein, T. P., F. E. Johnston, and L. Greinev. 1988. Energy expenditure and socio-economic status in Guatemala as measured by the doubly labelled water method. *American Journal of Clinical Nutrition* 47: 196-200.

Stephenson, L. S., ed. 1987a. *Impact of helminth infection on human nutrition*. London, New York, and Philadelphia: Taylor and Francis.

Stephenson, L. S. 1987b. Relations of S. hematobium, hookworm, and malarial infections and metrifonate treatment to nutritional status of Kenyan coastal schoolchildren. In *Impact of helminth infection on human nutrition*, ed. L. S. Stephenson. London, New York, and Philadelphia: Taylor and Francis.

Strauss, J., and D. Thomas. 1990. *The shape of the expenditure- calorie curve*. Discussion Paper Series. New Haven, Conn., U.S.A.: Institute of Economic Growth, Yale University.

Strauss, J., I. Singh, and L. Squire. 1986. *Agricultural household models: Extensions, applications, and policy*. Baltimore, Md., U.S.A.: Johns Hopkins University Press.

Strickland, S. S., and S. J. Ulijaszek. 1990. Energetic cost of standard activities in Gurkha and British soldiers. *Annals of Human Biology* 17: 133-144.

Stunkard, A. J., and I. Singh. 1972. Influence of social class on obesity and thinness in children. *Journal of the American Medical Association* 221 (6).

Sukhatme, P. V. 1961. The world's hunger and future needs in food supplies. *Journal of the Royal Statistical Society* A, 124.

Sukhatme, P., and W. Edmundson. 1989. Limits to nutritional adaptability. In *Abstracts of Fourteenth Meeting of the International Congress of Nutrition*, 527. Seoul: Secretariat, Department of Food and Nutrition, Ewha Woman's University.

Sukhatme, P., and S. Margen. 1978. Models for protein deficiency. *American Journal of Clinical Nutrition* 31: 1237-1256.

————. 1982. Autoregulatory homeostatic nature of energy balance. *American Journal of Clinical Nutrition* 35: 355-367.

Suzuki, S. 1959. Basal metabolism in the Japanese population. *World Review of Nutrition and Dietetics* 1: 103-124.

Svedberg, P. 1989. Undernutrition in Africa: Is there a sex bias? Institute for International Economic Studies, Stockholm. Mimeo.

Tanner, J. M. 1964. Human growth and constitution. In *Human Biology*, ed. G. A. Harrison, J. S. Weiner, J. M. Tanner, and N. A. Barnicot. Oxford, U.K.: Clarendon Press.

Teokul, W., P. Payne, and A. Dugdale. 1986. Seasonal variations in nutritional status in rural areas of developing countries: A review of the literature. *Food and Nutrition Bulletin* 8 (4): 7-10.

Thomson, A. M., F. E. Hytten, and W. Z. Billewicz. 1970. The energy cost of human lactation. *British Journal of Nutrition* 24: 565-574.

Tomkins, A. 1981. Nutritional status and severity of diarrhoea among pre-school children in rural Nigeria. *Lancet*: 860-862.

Tomkins, A., and F. Watson. 1989. *Malnutrition and infection*. ACC/SCN State-of-the Art Series: Nutrition Policy Discussion Paper No. 5. Geneva: Administrative Committee on Coordination/Sub-Committee on Nutrition.

Tonnies, F. 1937. *Community and society*. Trans. and ed. C. B. Loomis. East Lansing, Mich., U.S.A.: Michigan State University Press.

Torún, B., and F. E. Viteri. 1981. Energy requirements of preschool children and effects of varying energy intakes on protein metabolism. In *Protein-energy requirements of developing countries: Evaluation of new data*, ed. B. Torún, V. R. Young, and W. M. Rand, 229-241. Tokyo: United Nations University.

Valenzuela, M. 1988. Infant-mother attachment, child development, and quality of home care in young chronically undernourished children. In *Annual report 1988*. Lausanne, Switzerland: Nestlé Foundation.

Vasquez-Velasquez, L., A. M. Prentice, and A. W. Coward. 1989. Metabolic adaptation to negative energy balance in children. In *Abstracts of Fourteenth Meeting of the International Congress of Nutrition*, 421. Seoul: Secretariat, Department of Food and Nutrition, Ewha Woman's University.

Viegas, O. A. C., P. H. Scott, T. J. Cole, P. Eaton, P. G. Needham, and B. A. Wharton. 1982. Dietary protein energy supplementation of pregnant Asian mothers at Sorrento, Birmingham, Part II. *British Medical Journal* 285: 592-595.

Viteri, F. E. 1971. Considerations on the effect of nutrition on body composition and physical working capacity of young Guatemalan adults. In *Amino acid fortification of protein foods*, ed. N. S. Scrimshaw and A. M. Altschul. Cambridge, Mass., U.S.A.: MIT Press.

Viteri, F., B. Torun, M. Immink, and R. Flores, R. 1981. Marginal malnutrition and working capacity. In *Nutrition in health and disease and international development*, ed. A. Harper and G. Davis. New York: Liss.

Vosti, S. 1984. Nutrition, health and wages in rural South India. Ph.D. diss., University of Pennsylvania, Philadelphia, Pa., U.S.A.

Waaler, H. Th. 1984. Height, weight and mortality: The Norwegian experience. *Acta Medica Scandinavica* (Supplementum 679). Stockholm, Sweden.

Wade, J. W., M. M. Marbut, and J. M. Round. 1990. Muscle fibre type and aetiology of obesity. *Lancet* 335: 805-808.

Walker, T. 1984. Fluctuations in income in three villages of India's semi-arid tropics. International Crops Research Institute for the Semi-Arid Tropics, Patancheru, Andhra Pradesh, India. Mimeo.

Wandel, M., and G. Holmboe-Ottesen. 1992. Food availability and nutrition in regional perspective: A study for the Rukara region in Tanzania. *Human Geography* 20 (1): 89-107.

Waterlow, J. C. 1985. What do we mean by adaptation? In *Nutritional adaptation in man*, ed. K. Blaxter and J. Waterlow, 1-11. London: Libbey.

————. 1989. Nutritional adaptation: Responses to low intakes of energy and protein. London School of Hygiene and Tropical Medicine, London. Mimeo.

134

Watts, M. 1983. *Silent violence: Food, famine and peasantry in northern Nigeria.* Berkeley, Calif., U.S.A.: University of California Press.

World Bank. 1984. *World development report.* Washington, D.C.: World Bank.

Zeitlin, M. F., M. Mansour, and J. Bajrai. 1987. Positive deviance in nutrition: An approach to health whose time has come. In *Advances in international maternal and child health,* vol. 7, ed. D. A. Jelliffe. Oxford, U.K.: Clarendon Press.

Philip Payne is emeritus professor of applied nutrition at the London School of Hygiene and Tropical Medicine, U.K. Michael Lipton is professor of development economics at the School of African and Asian Studies, University of Sussex, Brighton, U.K., and was formerly director of the Food Consumption and Nutrition Policy Program at IFPRI. Richard Longhurst is an associate of The Institute of Development Studies and was formerly with the Ford Foundation in Khartoum, Sudan. James North is an economist at the Center for Naval Analyses, Alexandria, Virginia, and was formerly an intern at IFPRI. Steven Treagust was a research assistant at the Institute of Development Studies.